Scripts
and
Strategies
in
Hypnotherapy
Volume I

Roger P. Allen Dp Hyp PsyV

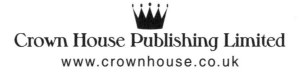

Crown House Publishing Limited
www.crownhouse.co.uk

First published by

Crown House Publishing Ltd
Crown Buildings, Bancyfelin, Carmarthen, Wales, SA33 5ND, UK
www.crownhouse.co.uk

and

Crown House Publishing Ltd
P.O. Box 2223, Williston, VT 05495-2223, USA
www.CHPUS.com

First published 1997
First paperback edition 2000
Reprinted 2001, 2002

British Library of Cataloguing-in-Publication Data
A catalogue entry for this book is available from the British Library.

ISBN 1899836462

Library of Congress Control Number 2002115603

Printed and bound in the UK by
The Cromwell Press
Trowbridge
Wiltshire

Dedication

I dedicate this work to my wife, Jill, with thanks
for love and understanding beyond measure.

Table of Contents

Acknowledgements

I find myself wishing fervently that I could remember each and every source of inspiration used within these pages. I have gleaned so much from the talks and seminars which I have attended, videos I have watched, tapes I have listened to, and, of course, from general conversations with others in the profession. I have no intention of making any claim to the many concepts in this book, or to indulge in any pretence that the ideas used in these scripts are anything other than an amalgamation of the products of many people's efforts which have become part of universal knowledge now.

The following is an honest attempt on my part to give credit where credit is due, and perhaps even to acknowledge that much of what I might call my own is but my own interpretation of ideas and thoughts coupled with experience shaped and coloured by the input of others before me - those whose influences have become a part of my therapeutic aim of helping those who come to us seeking help.

I have certainly been influenced by the late great master, Dr. Milton H. Erickson M.D., as, I would suggest, have so many before me. A special mention must be made of Bandler and Grinder, Steve and Connirae Andreas, Havers and Walters, Citrenbaum, King and Cohen, all of whom have figured greatly in my reading.

My approach in general within the book has been to give specific credit when I have been sure of the source. If I do not accurately record a source of inspiration, I would hope to be forgiven; my intention is honourable.

To all of those who have helped me with suggestions for scripts and with so much material, I express my heartfelt thanks and feel sure that those who will use the contents of this book will do so fully within the spirit in which it was submitted.

To Michael Carr-Jones and Tony Powell, I give special thanks for their unfailing positivity and encouragement.

Foreword

I expect that in most cases you, the reader, will be a new and beginning hypnotherapist. I remember well those very early days, when I sat nervously awaiting my very first paying client. On the wall hung my newly acquired diploma, and how conscious I was of the date upon that piece of paper! I had purposely hung it in a position where it could not be seen by clients other than when they first walked through the door. When sitting in my therapy chair, it was well situated within the far limits of peripheral vision.

My first client was a smoker, and, when he walked into the office, I noticed immediately that he was extremely nervous. I hoped that I was succeeding in my attempt to appear the confident professional, and that he would not pick up on the fact that I was quietly terrified.

The session went extremely well. After asking the relevant questions to discover his motivations and fears, his values and what was important to him, I then asked him to make himself comfortable and proceeded to induce hypnosis.

I used a script for smoking cessation that had been supplied by my teacher and mentor, Michael Carr-Jones, and, at the end of the session, I collected my first fee. I heard some months later that my first client was still not smoking, this information relayed to me from a client referred to me by him.

As time has allowed me to grow more confident in what I do, I have begun to realise that, although much therapeutic intervention is derived from the reactions of our own subconscious response to the client, the value of scripted material is important as it provides the framework for so many of my sessions.

Much of what I use is material which I have read in magazines and books, ideas picked up from seminars and simply ideas from the work of other therapists. I take these ideas and write them down so that now I have a database of scripted material and strategies that I can refer to whenever I am planning a therapy session.

It has been established in various schools that students who are using scripts in induction procedures invariably achieve better results. To begin with, the use of a script to induce hypnosis may appear somewhat constrictive, rather like building up a model from a pre-formed kit of parts. No imagination is needed: you just follow instructions and at the end you have your model airplane or whatever. In time you will develop a "feel" for the manner in which the scripts are structured and, as your confidence grows, you will venture beyond the framework and begin to add to it from your own unconscious resources.

You will find, for example, that the framework of the script which I have provided for smoking cessation can be modified for many other habit problems, as the verbiage becomes for you the tools of your trade that you can use in whatever way is effective and appropriate. As a developing hypnotherapist, you will evolve for yourself a style that you are comfortable with, as you move forward from within the guidelines that allow you to take those first tentative steps to becoming the effective therapist that you aim to be.

I make no apology for the fact that the scripts I have provided here will in some cases prove very similar to others that you may acquire from other sources. The reason I include them is that they meet the need, and in all respects the work that I have done in writing scripts for myself has to be recognized as an amalgamation of ideas. I will of course claim, and trust that you, the reader, will accept, that much of the material has incorporated within it a great deal of myself and my own responses to the problems that I have encountered.

This book is the product of many hours of dedicated and detailed work. It also includes the thoughts and ideas of a multitude of people, all utilized by me to construct what for me has been an invaluable basis for the therapy work that I so much enjoy.

It is for you to determine the value of my efforts, and I trust that the contents of this book will serve you well. Your comments, suggestions and questions are cordially invited, as you will no doubt make your contribution to the wealth of ideas that ensure that this great profession moves ever forward.

Roger P. Allen

Introduction

By way of introducing this work which contains much of that which is necessary to begin therapeutic practice utilising the medium of hypnosis, I feel that it is necessary to define in broad terms the elements that will be covered.

So much has been written concerning the "state" that is termed hypnosis and the attempts to describe it in scientific terms have been many. For the purposes of this book, I would describe the "state" of hypnosis as an altered "state" of awareness that will allow access to the subconscious, having reduced the critical analytical interference of the conscious rationalising processes.

The process of inducing hypnosis is in effect a focusing of the conscious processes to a point where an altered "state" of awareness is achieved. In this "state", those activities can be relaxed to the point where we still "hear", as our normal physical abilities are not impaired. This is similar to being engrossed in a television programme, whilst overhearing a conversation in the background.

Basically, all else just fades into unimportance. "There are three main components of the process of inducing hypnosis: relaxation, imagination, and enactment."   **Hildegard & LeBaron, 1984**

The subconscious part of the mind continues to hear all that is to be heard and in the same manner continues to react to stimuli whether visual, tactile, oral, olfactory, but is not subject to the same degree of rational conscious processing. The subject is not asleep or unconscious.

Information presented to the subconscious within this "state" will not be subject to the alterations of perception that are the mark of conscious processing of information and stimuli.

In stage hypnosis, this concept is often demonstrated by a suggestion such as that an onion given to the subject is in fact a juicy apple. The subconscious will accept the suggestion uninfluenced by the rational conscious mind. The subject will taste not an onion, but an apple.

Once trance "state" has been induced, then a process of deepening can be utilised, relaxing even more the constant chatter of the inner mind, allowing for therapeutic change to take place at a subconscious level.

Examples of deepening techniques are included in these pages. These techniques can be a very simple utilisation of a technique known as "compounding". Typical examples of this are: "as you experience X you can go ten times deeper into trance"; "I'm now going to take your right hand and, as I release it, it will fall into your lap just like a wet towel and you will go five times deeper into trance".

In order that we can facilitate changes in attitudes and behaviours, the therapeutic session continues using strategies that, when employed in conjunction with hypnosis, emulate recognised learning patterns. Suggestion therapy is very powerful, using positive affirmations that provide new and more beneficial responses to situations and conditions.

The practice of couching meaningful messages within metaphors was widely employed by the father of modern clinical hypnosis, Dr Milton Erickson. He used this technique as further distraction of conscious rationalisation while the important new learning was assimilated at a subconscious level. Hypnotherapy is in fact a teaching process, as we utilise the capabilities and the potential of the subconscious, taking advantage of our ever-increasing knowledge of learning patterns.

Whichever of the strategies is employed, they all have value and are effective. It is the skill and experience of the therapist in deciding which of the tactics available are most appropriate for his/her clients which will determine efficacy.

The hypnotherapy session concludes with a reorientation to conscious awareness, usually with a count. "I am now going to count from one to five and on the count of five you will be fully awake and aware". Of course, there is here an opportunity to give some suggestions such as: "On the count of five you will be fully awake and aware, feeling relaxed and comfortable as if you have had a refreshing nap". Discussion of the content of the therapy session is discouraged with the use of distractions such as, "What have you planned for the rest of the day?"

Within the scripts and strategies, I have included some italicised text. These items are for the guidance of the reader in his/her use in therapy, and I trust that these and the manner in which the material is presented will allow for easy understanding and utilisation.

A number of the scripts and strategies employ Neuro-Linguistic Programming (NLP) techniques. I would recommend that the reader take the opportunity to obtain some of the excellent works by Bandler & Grinder and by Andreas & Andreas on these concepts. I have included some of their works in the acknowledgements (at the end of this book), and they are available from most good book stores, or from the publishers of this book.

Inducing Hypnosis

It is my own belief that everyone can be hypnotized or, to be more accurate, that everyone is capable of attaining a state that we recognize as hypnosis. Much has been written by many learned theorists describing what is the hypnotic state, and I do not intend to allow myself to become embroiled in that particular debate. As a therapist I content myself with the fact that my clients are able to achieve a state that I am happy to describe as hypnosis, and that its use is of immense benefit as an adjunct to therapy. Entering this state is a natural ability that we all have, and we use it every day of our lives to enable us to focus attention.

When a first-time client is sitting in your consulting room, he/she will have brought to that session some preconceived ideas about hypnosis and those who use it in practice. In the main, their perceptions will probably have been shaped by the experience of watching a stage show. I find that it is always good practice to explore the perceptions of my clients to allay some of the fears that are usually present as a result of their experience.

"Will I be asleep?" I explain that they will be fully awake and fully conscious of everything that I say. "You will be very relaxed and comfortable and in effect the exact meaning of everything that I say to you will not concern you." I may then give an example as to how they have experienced hypnosis before, either by using the example of the television set and how everything else just fades into unimportance, or the example of the motorway journey when, having travelled at speed for some distance, there is a sudden realization that the conscious mind has not been fully involved in the driving. I'm sure that you will think of many similar examples that you can use.

"Will I do everything you tell me to do?" This should be recognized as the client's expression of their concern that they will not be in control, and that in some way you, the therapist, will have power over them. This is easily dealt with: I explain to my clients that they will be in complete control and that, if I were to suggest to them that they do something not within the realms of their normal moral code, either dangerous, illegal, or fattening, then quite simply they would not do it. Metaphors are always useful, and I often tell the story of how I went to see my bank manager in order to obtain funds for a particular project and how, having succumbed to my powers, he led me to the vaults telling me to just help myself. The point is usually effectively made!

Most of the questions are centred around this fear of losing control and so easily dealt with. It has to be sheer folly not to allow just a few minutes of the initial session to deal with this: it can save a lot of time later.

My usual preamble is contrived. I want that person sitting there in my therapy chair to accept my suggestions from the very outset. Just a small consideration will avoid the problem that so many call "resistance". "Okay Mary, what I would like you to do is make yourself very comfortable in that chair. Now would you prefer to go into hypnosis with your hands resting on a cushion in your lap or just resting on the arms of the chair?" (*Double bind*) "Now I realise that you will probably be wondering whether or not you will be able to go into hypnosis. If you just follow the simple instructions that I am going to give you, there is no way you can fail. Of course, you can resist me, but then that's not what you came for, is it?" In this way you will have established the rapport with your client that assures you of their compliance. Try it!

The first thing to do now is to achieve eye closure, and there are a few ways that you can do this. You can quite simply ask the client to close his/her eyes, but I myself prefer them to do it in their own time, with the thought that they are doing it because they want to go along with my suggestions.

I ask the client to look at a spot on my hand as I hold it just above their normal line of sight so that they have to strain their eyes upwards.

Eye Closure

"Now Mary, I want you to just pick a spot on the palm of my hand and just focus your eyes on that spot. You may notice that it is rather uncomfortable focusing your eyes on that spot and that it would be so nice to just close them, but I really don't want you not to close your eyes too quickly. You may notice how quickly your eyes begin to tire and become heavy, but that is fine; just focus on that spot as you listen to the sound of my voice. Nothing bothers you or disturbs you now as you listen to the sound of my voice, and the words that I say relax you .... and as I bring my hand down past your eyes you can follow that hand down past your nose...down past your mouth .... down under your chin, allowing them to close quite naturally .... closing now .... closing .... closing .... and that's fine .... I wouldn't want you to know now how much more comfortable you can feel as your eyes relax and you relax, completely in control now as you allow my words to just wash over you, each word relaxing you more and more."

(To continue, go to appropriate induction)

From this point on, it does not matter if you are reading from a script. After all, your client's eyes are closed and he/she cannot see what you are doing. Very soon now, as the trance state continues, they will not be concerned one jot, just comfortably relaxed. However, do not ignore your client: make sure you keep one eye on them to ensure that all is going well with them.

Voice modulation is important, and it can be very difficult to explain just how to deliver a hypnotic induction. I have used "...." to indicate pauses in the text, and would suggest that if you speak in a manner which is flowing and soft, reducing the speed of your delivery to about 70% of your normal speech rate, then you will not go too far amiss. Experience and practice will of course make perfect.

The technique above is the one that I use most frequently with my clients. However, there are many other techniques designed to achieve rapid eye closure which are equally effective. Some of these techniques have specific application such as working with children or anxious clients. There follows a number of these, as well as a technique for obtaining self-hypnosis.

Two Finger Eye Closure

An induction for adults:

Now (*client's name*), ... Take a long deep breath .... now just open your eyes wide, looking upwards towards your eyebrows, without straining your neck .... Now I am going to pull down your eyelids ... shut .... like this (use thumb and forefinger to gently close the eyelids). Now I want you to relax those muscles right there under my fingers .... just allow them to relax .... Relax them to the point where they just do not want to work .... and when you are sure that you have done that for yourself .... relaxed those muscles completely to the point where they just will not work .... then satisfy yourself .... have a try and find your eyes locking tighter and tighter .... (wait about 3 to 4 seconds.) .... That's fine .... there is no need to test them any further. Now you can allow that feeling .... that relaxation, to flow down through your body .... relaxing every muscle ... every fibre ... all the way down to the tips of your toes.

I am going to lift up your right hand now ... and shake, gently shake, relaxation into that hand ... that arm ... and when I release that arm, it will fall back into your lap just like a wet towel ... and you will go ten times deeper into relaxation. (Repeat with left arm.)

I have found this technique to be very effective when dealing with a sceptical client. It provides the client with proof that they have entered a trance state by not being able to open their eyes. The arm-drop test also provides an excellent deepening technique.

Children Up To The Age Of 10

(Begin in a conversational manner; it may help if you can find out what is the child's favourite toy.)

Now John, ... I expect that you play a lot with your toys at home .... I bet that you have a lot of toys and that when you play with them you pretend that they are real .... don't you ? .... I know that I did, when I was a little boy like you. Well .... you know we have a game of pretend here too .... and if you learn this game with me ... nothing that will happen here today will bother you at all. Would you like to learn this game? I'm sure you would.

Okay now John, ... let's start by taking a big deep breath in .... and then let it all out .... Now you can open your eyes just as wide as you can and I am going to show you this game of pretend. Now I am going to pull your eyelids closed .... like this .... (*Finger & thumb technique*) and you can pretend that you just can't open your eyes .... that's all you have to do .... just pretend as hard as you can that you just can't open your eyes no matter what .... pretend so hard that when you try to open your eyes ... they just won't work at all .... now try to make them work when you are pretending like that .... the more you try, the more they will not work because you are pretending so hard .... and because you are so good at pretending. Nothing that happens now will bother you or disturb you at all .... in your mind, you can be at home playing with your favourite toys ... and you need not concern yourself with anything else at all ....

Concept : David Elman

Fractional Induction

A general purpose induction:

As you rest so quietly there, just listening to the sound of my voice, I would like you now to concentrate on your feet and your toes. Concentrate on the muscles of your feet and feel any tension there in those muscles .... hold that tension .... and now just let it go .... allowing those muscles to soften and to loosen as you relax those muscles completely, letting go of tension .... letting go of anxiety now.

Now concentrate on the muscles of your ankles .... your calves and your knees, becoming aware now of the tension in those muscles .... feel that tension there .... hold that tension .... and now just let it all go .... allowing those muscles to soften and to loosen .... relaxing .... releasing .... just letting go as you listen to the sounds of my voice .... nothing bothers you or concerns you .... each word that I utter is just a signal for you to relax and go deeper .... and, as you go deeper now, you can become aware of the large muscles of your thighs .... feel the tension in those muscles .... feel the tightness here and then just let it go .... those large muscles softening .... loosening .... lengthening, as all the tension just drains away now .... as relaxation continues .... If you have done this correctly, you will become aware of that comfortable heaviness as your legs relax.

Now allow that heaviness and relaxation to move into the muscles of your buttocks and your pelvic region, all tension draining down now like the fine black sand in an hour-glass .... down into the bottom of the glass .... the passing of time .... time to relax and allow those comfortable feelings to continue as those muscles release all tension .... soften .... lengthen and loosen, and you drift deeper and deeper as my voice drifts with you now.

Now become aware of the muscles of your stomach and of your lower back .... feel the tension in those muscles .... and as you release that tension and those muscles relax .... soften .... lengthen .... loosen, you go deeper still as your body relaxes and your mind relaxes with it into peace and tranquillity, but now I really wouldn't want you to relax too quickly .... it's so much easier for you to allow that feeling to continue as you listen to the sounds of my voice .... the sounds in the room, and you can recognize that ability that is yours, to relax, and to reflect on your problems in a certain way.

Aware now of those muscles in your chest and your back .... aware of your breathing .... aware now of how relaxed and how quiet your breathing has become .... with each gentle breath you breathe out tension .... breathe out anxiety .... then breathe in peace .... harmony .... a feeling of security as muscles release their tension .... softening and loosening as you drift ever deeper .... feeling so comfortable and so good.

Now become aware of the muscles of your arms your hands, your shoulders, as you allow that relaxation to continue, relaxing each muscle, releasing tension, that comfortable heaviness continuing now, and it really can seem now to be too much effort to try even to make the effort to move those arms that are so heavy now as you listen to that voice speaking to you in soothing tones that relax you even deeper. Now the muscles of your neck .... feel the tension here .... now let it go and feel your neck shorten, as those muscles soften .... lengthen .... loosen .... all tension draining away now as your conscious mind becomes more and more comfortable and your unconscious mind assumes more and more of the responsibility for guiding and directing your thoughts .... your responses, as you allow this trance to continue.

Now become aware of the muscles of your face .... your jaw .... allow those muscles to just sag now as you release all of that tension .... your teeth slightly apart .... you feel the tip of your tongue now just brushing the back of your teeth as you drift still deeper .... relaxing .... releasing .... just letting go completely.

That feeling of relaxation can continue now into the muscles of your scalp .... the furrows of your forehead smooth over now as all tension just drains away and your entire body relaxes .... drifting in space .... that free floating place of effortless letting go as you now begin to use this opportunity to learn even more about your ability to relax .... and to let go completely .... as you drift into this trance more and more deeply .... more and more effortlessly .... and I continue to talk to you.

You can judge at this point whether you need to use a deepener script or continue with the session as you have planned.

Experience Induction

This induction is appropriate for anxious clients. Contra-indication: clients who have a fear of water.

Now you are resting comfortably THERE, listening to the sound of my voice HERE, with your eyes closed comfortably, you can be aware of your eyes and of how you are in control .... and how you could open them should you wish .... and that's fine, because I really wouldn't want you to not go into hypnosis too quickly, I would prefer that you discover how much easier it is simply to allow events to occur in their own time and in their own way .... and as you allow that feeling to continue in a shoulder .... a leg .... a hand, as you continue to listen to the sound of my voice .... the sounds that surround you .... the ticking of the clock perhaps or the distant murmur of traffic .... paying close attention now to those feelings .... those changes as they occur, as you wonder at your own ability to let go completely and drift into a trance, while your conscious mind has already begun to drift off somewhere else .... allowing the body to relax and the mind to relax .... without knowing at all how much more comfortable and relaxed you can become.

I wonder if you can remember now those experiences of drifting off whilst sitting comfortably watching television .... so engrossed in the story line .... listening to the voices as your eyes closed to rest quietly for a moment in time .... hearing the music .... or those words spoken .... in that quiet and relaxed way ... when a word or a sound brings to mind a particular memory .... and you drift into that memory .... dream away for a time .... come back to the words again .... until the words and the music become a soothing murmur .... a relaxing sound .... heard only in the background of the mind .... like a conversation overheard .... a peaceful and quiet time .... and the subconscious part of your mind continues to hear all that is important to you .... whilst your conscious mind drifts off to another place without really noticing that there is no need for you to make the effort to try .... to hear .... or to understand everything that is said or not said HERE .... as you rest so quietly .... THERE. You really have known all along how much easier it is to learn when you are so relaxed .... though I wouldn't want you to relax too quickly at first .... I would prefer that you discover now how much easier it is to recognize the small changes .... tiny changes .... almost imperceptible changes .... happening in your breathing .... and in your pulse .... how quiet and comfortable you have become as that feeling of security relaxes you even deeper than before. Your unconscious may choose to relax just one of your fingers before it continues to relax one of your thumbs .... or perhaps it will discover that your wrist will be a handier place to begin relaxing, but the conscious of your mind can enjoy being curious about exactly where those feelings will begin.

And now (*client's name*), please consider a stone being skipped across the clear calm surface of a pond .... the stone skips once .... twice .... three times and more .... each time the intervals shorter as it loses momentum .... slowing .... down more and more .... As it strikes the surface the peace and tranquillity is disturbed .... the water flows in ripples that spread in perfect rings .... but then the stone can skip no more .... all momentum is dissipated, its power lost .... and so it slips quietly down beneath the surface .... gently floating down .... past the creatures that live here .... drifting down .... gently ... quietly .... past the water plants .... and nothing is disturbed as it finally comes to rest there .... still now on the bottom of the tranquil pool .... and on the surface .... even the ripples become quieter as they spread in ever increasing circles .... to disappear entirely as the surface becomes calm again, and you can take the opportunity to quietly reflect upon those problems as you recognize now that ability that is yours .... to relax .... to let go of tension .... anxiety .... aware now of your ability to see things in a different way .... and to accept those things that seemed to be one thing and then turn out to be something else entirely .... and then the difficulty and ease that can be your experience, telling the difference between souls and soles .... sun and son .... bear and bare .... changing old beliefs .... recognizing new capabilities and capacities .... learning new ways of doing things.

I wonder now if you can allow those feelings to continue .... the same .... or to deepen even more now as you try to remember all those things I have said here .... about that pool there .... that television .... that stone that drifted down slowly .... even as you drift with your own thoughts .... and enjoy allowing that pleasant and comfortable experience of heaviness of arms .... of legs .... to continue there now as I continue to talk to you .... each word that I speak .... relaxing you deeper still.

You can judge at this point whether you need to use a deepener script or continue with the session as you have planned.

Question Of Reality

An induction to dissociate and observe reality:

I wonder if you have considered .... how to judge what's real ....

How do you make sense of it all?

Is it by what you see? .... That part that you consciously see?

Is it by what you hear with your ears? .... That part that you consciously hear?

And what you can feel with your touch? .... That part which you consciously know you are touching?

Or do you realise reality by the sense your subconscious makes?

Those feelings you feel on the inside?

Those sounds from within .... to you .... from you?

Those pictures in your mind?

Does your right hand know what your left hand is doing?

How do you create what is real?

And .... how else could you do that?

How many other flavours to reality do you think there might be .... which you can add to what you already taste? .... And .... which works best for you, and when?

You know, by how comfortable you feel.

Like a prism turning a single ray of light .... to a rainbow of colour .... your imagination is a prism for experience .... both past and future .... through which to perceive your present .... ponder your past .... anticipate your future.

And since it is your imagination, your senses can to create what is so.

So what would you like to create? Or should it be "who"?

Knowing that you determine what you experience .... and .... the meaning of the outcome .... you can choose to perceive those things which you enjoy .... which make you feel comfortable .... and/or .... learn more effectively .... from experience, either past or present, or future.

Self-Hypnosis Training Script

"There is an old saying, "If you give a man a fish, you have given him a meal. If you teach him how to fish you have given him a livelihood.

"Teaching those whom you work with is a means for insuring that your clients can continue to work independently and grow in your absence."

Michael Yapko, 1990

And now as I speak to you .... I wonder if you can close your eyes and remember those experiences of hypnosis that you have had before .... how easy it became to relax with those words spoken to you .... soft, soothing words that allowed you to let go of tension .... let go of cares as you drifted with those words and with your own thoughts too .... but today I would like you to know that you have that capability to go into trance and to utilize that experience completely by yourself .... not needing to know more about how to allow this alteration to occur .... and you can do this at any time that you want to or need to .... to allow you to use the abilities that are there for you as they have always been .... there in your perfect unconscious mind that can do so many things for you.

All you need to do is concentrate now on all of the muscles of your face .... and screw up those muscles so tight .... closing your eyes so tight .... and then feel that tension there .... feel that tension in your jaw .... in the muscles of your neck .... in your shoulders .... that tension spreading right down through your arms to the very tips of your fingers .... I would like you to really feel that tension and be intensely aware of the tightness and the discomfort in those muscles .... now hold it .... hold that tension .... and now I want you to count to three, and on the count of three .... release that tension, let it go completely .... your eyes remaining shut comfortably as all of the tension in all of those muscles just flows away now .... begin to count now with me .... 1 .... 2 .... 3 (*match breathing count on outward breath*) .... R-E-L-A-X .... that's good .... very good ....·relaxing releasing .... letting go completely as every muscle relaxes and you drift down with that relaxation as it occurs .... allowing that comfortable heaviness to increase .... to flow down .... softening .... each muscle loosening as that relaxation increases now .... You can continue to drift down as you allow that trance to deepen now as you remember all that you experienced before .... that feeling of comfort .... of security perhaps .... as you relax each and every small part of you .... allowing the subconscious of your mind to accept the responsibility for taking care of those things that are important to you .... as your conscious mind drifts to wherever it wishes to .... perhaps to a special place that your subconscious will provide for you .... where you can relax even deeper .... secure .... safe .... enjoying that pleasant feeling of experiences of trance remembered .... where you can utilize those experiences that can help you .... and as you drift down .... then so you can drift back again .... in your own time as you choose when your attention is required or just when you want to .... drifting back to full wakeful awareness as your eyes open .... and you can take this opportunity to practise again your ability to create your own state of comfortable hypnosis .... creating that tension, as before .... feeling that tension, that discomfort .... and then .... counting to three .... to release that tension .... and allow that trance to develop and to continue .... as you allow that drifting down .... deeper and deeper .... each breath of yours relaxing you more .... that experience of yours continuing as you allow it to .... and I would like you to continue now to practise that ability .... to drift down .... to enjoy that experience and then to drift back again .... so go ahead now while I sit here quietly and wait for you .... that's very good.

(Allow a minute or two to elapse and then continue)

I am very impressed, *(client's name)*; you have learned very well how to do that for yourself .... how to create that tension .... and then to release that tension .... and to drift down into a comfortable state of self-hypnosis where you can utilize the abilities and capacities that your subconscious mind can provide for you .... that creative part of you, where those special capabilities and capacities will be available to you even more than before .... your subconscious mind can do so many things for you .... as you drift down into that trance in your own time and in your own way .... to ask that your unconscious provide those things needed for you .... aware that all that you need to do is to relax in that way .... and ask it to do so .... and then to drift back up again .... in your own time .... in your own way .... bringing with you those comfortable positive feelings of balance .... of things resolved .... feeling refreshed .... as you reach the surface of wakeful awareness .... allowing your eyes to open .... as you take a deep breath and smile.

Have your subject practise this procedure once or twice before leaving the office, and emphasis the need to practise this new skill for their own benefit during the whole of their life.

Deepeners:

The Candle

Now as you relax more, and let go more and more, you can allow every muscle in your body to relax.

Now picture in your mind, a candle .... this candle can be any colour you wish it to be. The colour that you have chosen for your candle is a colour that your subconscious knows relaxes you and calms your mind.

Now focus on the flame of the candle. See how beautiful the colours within the flame are. You may see red, blue, yellow, purple, white or maybe another colour, and as you see the colours within the flame, you relax more and go deeper, as you enjoy these heavy and relaxed feelings, these hypnotic feelings.

Now focus on the wax body of your candle. As you see the first trickle of melting wax, begin to move down the side of this warm and comfortable candle.

Now see the melting wax touch the candle holder and merge with it to become part of the candle holder .... You become more and more relaxed, safe and comfortable.

Now imagine that you are that candle, a candle of total relaxation and, as you picture it, as a particular muscle in your body, helping you to relax more and more completely. Picture the chair that you are sitting in, as a candle holder, and that your muscles, like the wax of your candle of relaxation, are melting into the chair and that you are becoming, yourself, a candle of relaxation.

Anon

A gentle deepener, ideal where a light trance is required.

The Mind's Eye

"In the same way that you have eyes that see the world around you, you also have an inner eye that we call "the mind's eye".... and it can see images and process thoughts even as you relax so deeply .... and the mind's eye has an eyelid and, like your physical eye, that eyelid can close down .... as it too becomes heavy and tired ... wanting to close .... and it can begin to close .... and, as it slowly drops, it shuts out stray thoughts .... stray images, and can leave your mind perfectly clear .... it experiences whatever you would choose .... and it's closing now .... closing more and more ... and you mind grows quiet and at peace .... and now it closes completely ... .. closing out all stray thoughts or images that you don't want to interfere with how relaxed you are ...."

Michael Yapko, 1990

An extremely effective technique, that can be utilized to "damp down" the continual internal self speak, allowing for deeper trance experience.

The Garden

As you go deeper now .... your subconscious mind becomes open .... more accessible and receptive to new learnings .... to changing old beliefs .... as you relax so comfortably there .... just listening to the sound of my voice .... here .... so calm .... a feeling of peace and tranquillity .... allows you to relax more and more .... with each easy breath .... with each gentle beat of your heart.

As I count down from ten to one .... you can just let go and you can go deeper now .... with each count .... using each number to let go of stress and tension .... to go deeper now.

Ten .... As you allow each muscle and nerve in your body to relax .... letting go .... becoming calm .... you feel peaceful .... comfortable now.

Nine .... You relax your mind and your body together .... and if you lose track of the progression of the numbers .... then that's fine .... just let go now .... as ....

Eight .... You start to sense a gentle connection between your mind and your body .... and an inner wisdom.

Seven .... Go deeper now .... and as you breathe out .... *(Start to pace with breathing)* .... start to breathe out fear .... breathing out anxiety now.

Six .... Letting fear .... anger and stress flow away from your body .... with every outward breath .... letting go now .... slowly .... comfortably .... calmly.

Five .... And now with each outward breath .... I want you to start saying a word to yourself .... without moving your mouth or your tongue .... your breathing not changing .... your throat perfectly still .... on each outward breath .... say the word inwardly to yourself .... CALM .... *(pace with outward breath, and repeat.)* .... CALM.

Four .... Without thinking what it means .... without analysing the word .... just moving the sound inward now .... so that it seems to come from an inner wisdom .... *(continue to match breathing)* .... CALM.

Three .... Gently now .... easily .... calmly .... calm .... letting go .... and whenever your mind strays from that sound .... and it will stray away .... then just acknowledge that fact and gently bring it back .... repeating to yourself the word .... CALM .... *(matching breathing)*.

Two .... Continuing now to relax .... and to let go .... gently drifting down .... into peace and harmony of body .... mind .... and spirit.

One .... And as you continue to drift deeper still .... you begin to see .... sense or imagine yourself in a beautiful garden .... the sun is shining .... gently warming your skin .... comfortable .... you look across the lawn as it sweeps away to an ornamental pond .... with a fountain playing .... the water droplets sparkling .... glistening .... in the soft, diffused light that filters down through the leaves and branches of the ancient trees that surround this garden .... shielding and sheltering this beautiful place.

The grass is soft .... springy beneath your feet, and as you walk .... you pass flower beds cut into the lawn .... filled with the most beautiful flowers and plants .... so many varieties and colours .... and you can be aware of the fragrance of the flowers carried to you on a soft breeze that drifts across the garden .... rustling the leaves .... causing the heads of the flowers to sway gently .... the subtle sound of nature all around .... birds singing .... the drone of insects and the splash and gurgle of cascading water .... each sound .... each sensation relaxing you more .... comforting as you drift deeper .... and every step becoming heavier.

You soon find yourself in a small clearing .... the sun warming you and relaxing you more and more now .... as you sit .... resting your back against a large and ancient tree .... the bark of the tree is soft and comfortable .... and you sense that many people have rested here as you are resting now .... but although you are alone .... you feel safe here .... peaceful .... comfortable .... the word CALM .... comforts you more as your mind drifts and fades.

This is perhaps one of the most frequently used deepeners in use. However before using this technique do check with your client first that they have no aversions to gardens or have problems with hay fever or similar allergies. If they do then use another more appropriate technique.

Continue with session as planned.

The Stair

Now you can allow your inner mind to show you standing at the top of a fine marble staircase, with ten steps leading down. There is a firm handrail and here you feel safe and secure .... nothing concerns you at all. In a moment you can walk down that staircase and as you hear me count off each of the steps, you can step down one step .... doubling your relaxation with each step you take.

Begin now as I count .... Ten .... Doubling your relaxation going deeper *(pace with breathing)* .... Nine .... Deeper still .... Eight .... Letting go of tension as you relax and go deeper. .... Seven .... Doubling your relaxation .... deeper still .... Six .... Aware now of your breathing and how comfortable it has become .... Five .... Each gentle breath relaxes you .... you relax more with each breath that you take .... Four .... Deeper .... even deeper into a state of profound relaxation of mind and body .... Three .... Doubling your relaxation going ever deeper .... Two .... The deeper you go, the better you feel .... and the better you feel, the deeper you go .... One .... Almost all the way down now into total relaxation .... Zero .... Now stepping off the bottom step and you can find yourself in a place that is comfortable and safe for you to be .... a place of safety and security where there is no anxiety .... no fear .... just tranquillity .... and calm peace.

This is a really effective technique favoured by many therapists. It is popular as it matches the internal state of the client and their rate of breathing to your words. Very occasionally you may find a client breathing increasingly more deeply with each count that you make. If this occurs just say "breathe comfortably, only as deeply as you need to relax even more deeply ...." and then return to counting.

Continue with session as planned

Suggestion Therapy:

Ideomotor Response
(I.M.R.)

There are many occasions in therapy where it is necessary to ask the client questions and to receive answers. It is a widely held belief that asking the client to speak can interfere with the depth of the trance. So, in order to avoid this, the client is asked to communicate via finger movements to signal yes or no. This technique is known as ideomotor response.

As you relax comfortably .... you can be aware of the fact that going deeply into hypnosis is a rewarding and pleasant experience, and that any discomfort that you may feel will only occur in the context of the therapy .... and only if I direct you to.

Now I want you allow yourself to go even deeper .... drifting down into a state of profound relaxation of mind and body .... sensing now a gentle connection between your mind .... your body and your innermost self. With each breath that you take you relax deeper into peace and calm .... tranquillity.

And now I want to speak to that part of you which is all-knowing .... knows all about (*client's name*) .... and forgets nothing .... and which never tells a lie.

I will from time to time be asking questions that require a yes or no answer .... you can answer me by allowing the pointing finger of your right hand to lift if the answer to my question is Yes. I will now touch that finger (Touch finger) .... If the answer to my question is No, then you can allow me to know by allowing the pointing finger of your left hand to lift. I will now touch that finger. (*Touch Finger.*) (*Repeat Paragraph*).

Should you not know the answer to my question, or wish not to divulge this to me, then you can indicate this to me by allowing both of the pointing fingers of your right and your left hand to lift simultaneously.

(*Client's name*) need know nothing of this as he/she communicates with me verbally, reporting to me those thoughts and feelings .... images .... events as are necessary for the purposes of this therapy.

Roger P. Allen

Do you understand the instructions that I have given to you? *(Watch for response)*.

Continue with session as planned.

Sports Performance

As you prepare to (*engage in or play sport*), allow your imagination to show you a scene, a familiar place perhaps, or one that you can create for yourself, it does not matter at all, as long as you can find this place restful and strengthening, a place where you would choose to be if you felt a bit low or depressed and you wanted to feel better.

If you wish, you can choose to have somebody there with you, someone special to you who makes you feel good, who gives you strength and purpose. This person may be a brother or a sister, mother or father or someone who is very close to you. It may be someone whom you admire from afar, living or otherwise. By doing this and allowing yourself to experience that place and that person, you are choosing a place and a person who strengthens and motivates you to your maximum potential.

Some can draw strength from a scene such as a candle flickering, a watermill turning, or a bonfire, or a mountain stream as it rushes over the rocks. It matters not, as long as it is a scene which provides for you an inner peace and tranquillity and gives to you a special feeling of confidence and inner strength of purpose.

So now (*client's name*) .... imagine yourself at that place and, at peace with your own inner self, or with that special person, and allow that special feeling of calm and confidence, of tranquillity of spirit to grow and to expand, as you experience it, breathe in the essence of it, breathe in the clear air, absorb the powerful and positive vibrations, and, with each breath, you can feel that strength and purpose, feel your mental and physical being strengthening.

Experience now that surge of energy pulsing through your body as your powers centralize, as your mind focuses intently on the task at hand, your concentration and your energies vibrating and pulsing with positive intent and purpose, your mind and body in perfect tune as you prepare for that moment when all of your energies physical and mental will integrate with the finely honed skills and techniques and burst forth in perfect harmony and unison, as your mind sees you completing the (*race, task, performance*) .... achieving your goal, a winner, a champion.

As you do this feel yourself gaining in strength and health, increasing your vitality, taking all that you need physically and mentally from this experience, feeling better and stronger, more alive, more confident in your ability to achieve, to win, to overcome.

Practise this for just a few minutes each and every day, actually drawing the strength and the vitality, both physically and mentally from whatever helps you. Know that you can do all that you need to do, whatever you want to do, whatever you believe you can do. You can do it, if you allow your mind to accept that you can do it. You can do anything that you want to do if you want it enough and you believe in your own abilities and capacities for greatness and for achievement.

Practise this and then practise some more, for a few minutes each and every day, practise to train your mind to give you the best opportunity and the positive belief in your ability to prevail. Once you have done that, you can relax, confident and assured in the knowledge that you have prepared yourself in the most effective and diligent way possible to be the best that you can be, the best that you can ask yourself to be. Know and believe that, if it is attainable, if it is realistic, then it is achievable, what your mind can conceive, it can achieve. Whatever you believe, you can achieve. Work on believing it and as you believe it it will be so and you will achieve.

When you are in competition, before you make a single move, you can visualize in your mind a successful outcome. Visualize what you wish to happen happening for you, what you need to do to do well, for you to succeed.

Practise doing this every day as part of your training and preparation, and never make a move when you are actually competing without visualizing a successful outcome. Concentrate on what will happen next, in the next few minutes or the next few seconds. What happened before does not concern you at all, it is of no value to you as you shut out from your mind all that is not important to you in your quest for excellence. Visualize with all your strength and concentrate on only that which is important, the present moment and the immediate future, on what will happen next. You will shut out all that is unimportant and irrelevant, concentrating on that special moment, as all of your abilities and strengths concentrate and unite in perfect harmony, providing for you the perfect balance of concentration, of positive tension and calmness and clarity of thought, your body and mind perfectly attuned to provide you with maximum and most effective concentration of effort both physically and mentally

You will concentrate on that future and concentrate on making it happen.

You have all that you need to perform at your very best and you know that you will perform to your highest potential. You have excellent powers of judgment, your decision-making will be at its optimum performance, you will be clear and definite, and in excellent form both mentally and physically, you will have all of the determination, confidence and the stamina to perform at your best and for as long as you need to in order to achieve your highest potential. You believe in yourself, believe in your ability, whatever you do you will do well and you will do it better than you have ever done it before. You now believe yourself to be a winner. You are a winner.

Pass Your Driving Test

..s you go deeper now .... each breath relaxing you more .... you can imagine it is time for you to demonstrate your ability and skills as a driver .... knowing that you are going to be successful. What usually occurs is that which you expect .... and you expect that you will be calm .... confident .... relaxed and in complete control. You expect that you will pass your test easily and without effort .... and you know now that what you thought could be difficult .... will be so very easy because you are relaxed and in the perfect frame of mind to succeed.

When you are called upon to demonstrate your skill as a driver you will be calm .... confident .... and completely relaxed.

You will be so pleasantly surprised at the ease with which you will maintain your calm and confident manner .... as you demonstrate your skills and your abilities as a driver .... you will be amazed that something you had thought would be difficult .... will be so very very easy .... it will be easy because you will be completely relaxed and calm .... and in this relaxed and calm .... confident state you will be in the perfect frame of mind .... you will be successful .... you will pass your driving test.

Now *(client's name)*, I want you to visualize as vividly as you can these following scenes that I will suggest to you. Every day .... I want you to practise visualizing these scenes .... imagine them as vividly as you can .... and in every scene you are calm .... confident .... and relaxed.

You are now in the car driving to the test centre. After completing the necessary formalities .... you emerge from the test centre with your examiner .... and you walk towards your car. You now sit in the car and make all of the necessary checks and adjustments before you start the engine.

Now you are driving the car and doing all of those things that you have learned .... you perform each and every stage of your driving extremely well. Imagine yourself .... carrying out a three point turn .... excellent .... Now reversing around a corner .... keeping just the right distance from the kerb .... perfectly ....

Now imagine yourself parking the car between two other vehicles .... taking your time .... judging the distance just right .... parking beautifully .... excellent.

Now imagine yourself performing an emergency stop .... braking the vehicle to a halt quickly and with complete safety .... perfectly.

Now imagine yourself doing a hill start .... balancing engine .... clutch and hand brake absolutely perfectly .... pulling way smoothly .... very good! Imagine yourself driving in traffic .... keeping a proper distance .... using your mirrors .... observing and giving proper consideration to all other road users .... driving safely and smoothly .... with anticipation and confidence .... knowing that you are competent and have studied and practised until you are perfect.

Practise visualizing these scenes as vividly as you can throughout the day as often as you can .... in the morning .... when settling down for the night .... whenever you have some time to yourself .... seeing yourself at all times .... calm .... confident .... and relaxed.

You have studied the Highway Code .... all of the information that you need is there in your memory because you have made the effort to study .... all of this information will spring instantly to mind and to your lips at the moment when you need it .... so see yourself right now .... answering questions on the Highway Code .... see yourself answering each question easily and fluently .... answering every question correctly .... and you expect to be right .... perfect!

Now imagine the examiner .... telling you that you have passed the test .... congratulating you .... handing you a piece of paper confirming that you are now a qualified driver.

When you actually take your test .... you will have taken your test so many times in your mind, it will be like something that you have done before many times .... with great skill and confidence .... in reality it will happen just as you have practised in your mind.

You will find it easy to produce a polished and accomplished demonstration of your driving skills .... You are going to pass your test .... you are going to pass your driving test with consummate ease.

You will be aware of a voice that speaks to you from within .... as you take your driving test .... you will hear the calm and comforting voice of the skillful driver within you .... that voice will calm you .... it will relax you.

Please practise your visualizations as many times as you can throughout your day .... visualize each and every step .... each action .... each procedure .... do it in the morning .... do it before you retire at night .... in every scene see yourself .... calm .... confident .... and relaxed .... skillful .... and knowledgeable.

You have done all that you need to pass your driving test .... you have prepared yourself physically .... you have practised all the skills and the techniques that are necessary .... you have the experience .... you have done it all many times successfully .... you have studied the Highway Code .... you are prepared mentally and physically .... just believe that you can pass and you will pass your driving test ....

Now go .... and pass your driving test.

Metaphors:

Emelda

This metaphor was written especially for Kay, a young lady of 28 years who was causing her now retired parents much distress through her ever increasing demands on them. The purpose of the therapy was to allow her to realise at a subconscious level that she was responsible for her own life and that her demands were unreasonable.

I am reminded of a story about a very wealthy landowner who many years ago was famous for his kindness and generosity to those who were in his service. He had many servants and retainers, and, for their benefit, he established a fine home where they could live in comfort and security in their old age.

He had two daughters of whom he was very proud as a father should be and doted on them both, giving to them all of his love, for he had lost his own wife, their mother, in childbirth when the younger daughter was born. The elder of the daughters was of a loving and kind disposition, taking after her father, and was soon married to a prince who took her far away.

The other daughter was a concern to her father who noted well her manner of always getting her own way through her disruptive behaviour and manipulative ways. But he loved her and in his concern for her he charged one of his most trusted servants and the servant's wife that they should take care of her and be responsible for her well-being on his death.

Although the daughter was not best loved by the servants, the man concerned gave his pledge to his master that he would indeed ensure that the rich man's daughter was looked after.

The rich man provided for the couple a generous income and a comfortable home across the valley so that they could live in comfort in return for their watching over the daughter and ensuring that no harm came to her.

Eventually the rich man died, and, as he had no son, his daughter inherited from him half of his wealth and the great manor house and all it contained. Now the work of the servant and his wife began. In her fashion, the daughter devised a complex manner of ensuring that the retainer and his wife would always be at her beck and call, for were they not responsible for her, had they not promised her father?

On the top of the mansion house walls, she caused to be installed a great drum and a huge horn, the beat and the note of which were such that they would fill the valley with her calls, and none would escape the noise of her demands. Also was erected here a large flag-pole from which she could fly banners which demanded the attention of the retainer and his wife.

Her calls were loud and many and her manner towards the faithful retainer and his wife became ever more abusive. But the promise to take on the responsibility for the daughter's well-being had been given by an honourable man. Without complaint he took from her the responsibility of her own well-being. Many were the times when he and his wife would trek across the valley to answer her calls, to draw the water from the well and to cut the wood for the fire, to cook and to clean as she wasted her life, lay in her bed, growing larger and less attractive to those who would woo her for her wealth, indulging herself at the expense of those who now loved her not as they had loved her father.

As the retainer and his wife grew older, so they became more frail and the work of their demanding mistress became too much. They asked for help, that their mistress might employ others to help them, but her reply was, "Whose responsibility is it to look after me?" They received no consideration at all. As the old man grew more frail and more slow, then the beating of the drum and the blast of the horn grew louder and more insistent, and all in the valley heard the clamour of her demands and kept away.

But the old retainer and his wife, ever faithful to their promise, struggled ever on to do their best. Slowly and painfully they kept to the task, now to be beaten for their slowness and abused with the lash of the woman's tongue for their failing strength. Those who ran the home for the elderly ex-servants of the rich man tried in vain to persuade them both to give up their charge, for they had done their duty, done their best and without gratitude or consideration.

"Come now and enjoy the retirement that you have earned, take on that responsibility which can only be yours, while you can still stand on your own two feet, and allow others to take on the responsibility which never was yours and can never be removed from that person who is responsible for that life." But the old man persevered, for he had given a pledge.

The day came when the drums were beating and the horn blasts filled the air with their demanding row, but the onset of age had dimmed the eyes and the hearing of the old couple, and for them the world was quiet and peaceful, time to enjoy the loving company that had been the mainstay of their marriage.

The daughter fumed and raged; the noise was horrendous, but to no avail. She called for her carriage and at a breakneck pace rode to the cottage where the old couple had lived at her beck and call for these many years. Her years of self-indulgence were apparent now, her gluttony immersing her former beauty within a now grotesque body, her face livid with rage and hatred at this unforgivable lapse in the attention to her whim. She crashed through the door. Within the old man dozed in the chair by the fire as his wife, now hobbling with the aid of a stick, busied herself with the preparation of their evening meal. Her rage was enormous as she lashed out with her cane, striking the old man from his chair, cursing the elderly couple with the language of the gutter as she set about them in her tantrum. Even though she recognized the frailty of those who had taken so much responsibility for her, she would show no consideration, and so she smashed and destroyed the things that were precious within that home, screaming her rage at the world. It was the coachman who saved them more hurt. He seized the struggling Emelda and threw her back into the coach. He then drove her back to the big house, and locked her in her room to allow her temper and rage to subside. He took care of the horses as he had done for so many years and then packed up his few possessions and left, never to return.

The home over the mountain had two new residents the following day, for those who were concerned came and they fetched the old couple away from harm. Now they would live the remainder of their lives in the peace and harmony they deserved, that responsibility so long misplaced now firmly laid where it belonged. They would enjoy the sunshine and the softening glow of eventide in the evening of their lives, looking not back at those years so cruelly taken from them, now responsible only for themselves, having done their best and more.

And what of the daughter? What happened to her? Who would care now? WHO WOULD TAKE RESPONSIBILITY FOR HER LIFE AND WELL-BEING NOW?

Perhaps she did make the effort to put aside old ways and to listen to that wise inner voice; perhaps she accepted the responsibility for her own life; perhaps she looked from within herself to others and thereby grew as a special and unique person, to become part of life as it is and to enjoy what there is.

I hope that she will be OKAY; I wonder what you think? WILL SHE BE OKAY?

Bicycles

This metaphor was written specifically for a young lady who had been with her fiancé for a number of years and was now finding herself attracted to another man at work. He was the complete opposite of her fiancé, extroverted and brash, devil-may-care. He had shown an interest in our heroine, but then he had shown an interest in so many others before. How was she to choose what was true reality?

As you relax more and more .... the mind can wander at times the way that nomads wander from place to place .... never going anywhere special, just drifting from here to there .... which can sound so romantic and so relaxing too .... unless there is something you want to do or somewhere that you want to go .... something that really is important for you to have .... because it really can be difficult to arrive at your goal if you do not know where you are going .... don't use a map, just take a turning to the right here .... and there a turn to the left .... to the right again without a plan .... and then wondering which is the right direction to go .... what do you really want to do?

Consider now the animals of this world .... those that migrate from place to place .... How would it feel if you were to wake one day and suddenly feel that feeling that tells you .... as sure as you can be, that it is time to do something different .... time to fly south .... time to swim north .... to cross the ocean .... or the mountains .... the feeling that the whales feel .... that the snow geese feel .... that the king salmon feels .... that the wildebeest feel.

I wonder how it would feel to know something without knowing why .... know something deep down .... and be so sure that you know .... what is wanted .... what is needed .... in the way that a small child knows when it needs to drink .... but still does not know what thirsty means .... a craving .... perhaps a desire .... wanting .... whenever our mind can picture the kind of meal that we crave.

You watch people in a restaurant .... looking through the menu .... allowing their mind to imagine the texture of this food or the taste of that .... until they find one that tastes perfect to the mind .... like trying on clothes to see if they suit .... or possible futures .... imagining the time and the place .... that tastes .... feels .... looks and sounds just right .... yes, that's it .... everything in imagination .... just fine .... experiencing that future feeling of satisfaction when everything is just fine .... and you finally have what is needed .... and have done all that is required to have that way of being you

.... to hold that wonderful feeling .... and to know that there is no need to wonder .... no need to wander any longer .... to know what direction to take and to enjoy that knowing and going there when you want to from now on .... like a homing pigeon that somehow seems to know which way there .... back to where it belongs .... it gets its bearings .... knows which way to go and it goes there to where it needs to be to feel comfortable and happy .... where it needs to be.

And I am reminded too of the man who rode a bicycle each and every day to his work and then back home in the evening .... a machine that he had had for many years .... a gift from someone who loved him .... someone who was happy to make him happy. He was so delighted with that bike .... he cleaned it and polished it .... oiled it and made certain that every small part was kept in good condition. The bicycle served him well .... carrying him so many hundreds of miles .... to work and even on holidays .... carrying too all of his camping equipment .... and all that he needed to enjoy the experience without concern that he would not have what was needed.

He called one day at a shop in town to buy a new tyre for his tried and tested steed .... and it was then that he saw the new model .... a bicycle with all of the newest features .... deraillier gears .... sports handlebars .... a drinks container that he could drink from as he rode .... the paint was so bright and so shiny .... and he wondered how it would be to ride that bike .... to own that bike .... after all, the one he had was old .... and he knew it so well .... all of its scratches .... all of its little faults .... things that needed to be attended to, like the tyre that was now worn .... and there was no desire .... no feeling of excitement .... at what was known .... so familiar .... and so he determined right there and then that that bicycle would be his .... that he would save all of his money and would have for himself that new and exciting machine.

He continued to ride his old bike .... now imagining himself on that new machine .... longing for the day when he would achieve his goal and own that new machine .... but he neglected his old bike that had carried him through .... and carried him still .... did not bother to clean it or to look after it any more .... as he dreamed only of that machine that would be his.

Then came the day when he realized that dream .... that new bike was his, and he abandoned his old and faithful machine .... leaving it to rust and decay in the garden shed of his parents' home .... and he rode that bike in all its splendour .... others admired it and wanted it too .... and then one day it was taken away .... stolen .... and he was so sad .... that attractive machine .... that so many others admired and desired .... had been taken by another .... never to be seen again.

He went back to that old and faithful machine .... and soon discovered that it had been there all the time .... there when he needed it .... ready to begin again .... and not to complain or let him down .... and he never ever did need to drink whilst riding along .... some attention now needed .... and a coat of paint can be so easily applied .... even as the imagination can choose to allow that look or this look to seem perfect or not .... and when that knot is tied .... will that knot be the one that will slip .... or not ....?

And I know that you too will choose that which is right for you to do .... aware of what is true and that which is durable .... that will be there whenever you need the comfort and the stability of something comfortable .... like a jumper or a pair of shoes that fits just so .... aware of the comfort .... and aware that you do not need to know how it is comfortable .... it does not concern you .... it is just comfortable .... as your own unconscious mind is allowed now to do those things .... that are the right things for you .... as you trust even more than ever before that part of you which takes care of your best interests .... to your highest good.

The Art Collection

Metaphor for smoking & substance abuse etc.

I am reminded of a man whom I new many years ago, named Henry, who was very interested in art. He didn't have much money, but he worked hard and saved what he could to put together a very fine collection of works of art of which he was justifiably proud.

He consulted an acquaintance of his, an acknowledged expert, as to the best way of looking after his collection of fine porcelain and china. The acquaintance sold him a special substance, which he had formulated, with precise instructions as to the manner and the frequency with which it should be used. He told Henry that, if he used it regularly, then he would have no need to worry and that he could just relax, happy in the knowledge that he was doing the best he could to preserve his collection of fine works.

Henry paid the money and, throughout the years, he cleaned and lavished attention on his valued collection, always ensuring that he purchased a good supply of the compound, feeling relaxed with the thought and the idea that he was doing the best that he could to ensure the well being of his works of art.

He failed to notice the fact that he always seemed to have a dull throbbing headache. The skin on his hands became reddened and sore, his fingernails became brittle and unsightly, and nothing seemed to make it better. He was unaware of the pungent smell that had become part of his person. It clung to his clothes and his hair. At least he had his collection of fine works of art.

It was a few years before he managed to put aside enough money to take the holiday that he had planned for so long. Before he left, he asked a very good friend of his to look after his collection while he was away. He gave precise instructions as to how the art treasures should be cleaned and attended to, using the special compound that was so important to him for his peace of mind. The friend promised to do as Henry asked, even though the smell of the compound was disgusting, and it so easily stained his hands and clothing.

Henry went on his holiday and was amazed to discover that after just a few days the headaches and the pains, the reddened and sore hands, cleared up and he felt so much better and more alive than he had felt for such a long time.

Imagine how he felt on his return when he found that his friend was unwell, suffering as he had done. And the smell now so apparent upon him was so disgusting. He quickly deduced that the compound that he had relied on so much for peace of mind was the problem, and a professional analysis established that it was full of poisonous and toxic chemicals. That very day Henry destroyed his whole stock of the compound, and he knew that his health was worth more than any possession no matter how valuable or rare. Henry sought further advice from the most respected experts in their field as to alternatives to meeting his responsibility of caring for his all-important works of art, in a beneficial and healthy manner.

To his surprise, the answer was simple and inexpensive, and it had been there in front of him all the time: simple solutions of mild and appropriate cleaning materials would achieve exactly the results that he desired. His works of art would be cleaned and cared for in the most natural way that would prove healthy and beneficial.

The manufacturer of the compound would continue to produce and sell his lethal poison without regard or pity for those who would suffer from his irresponsible and mercenary actions, but Henry had made the decision to take responsibility for his own life and his own health. No longer would he rely on the advice of others whose best interests were not Henry's. He had accepted the evidence as it was, relying on his own judgment and his own ability, not knowing or needing to know how his own inner mind knew what to do for him, and I wonder now if you will not now allow your own wise inner advisor to do those things needed for you? .... and you will, will you not?

*(Go to **Stop Smoking** or whichever script is appropriate.)*

The above metaphor lends itself to so many applications. I wonder how many you will find it useful for?

Anchors

An anchor is simply a stimulus which initiates a response, in the same way that you will experience some anxiety perhaps whilst in the waiting room of your dentist, or that funny feeling you get when you see a police car in your rear view mirror, and that response of glancing at the speedometer.

Then, of course, there is the subconscious stimulus that results in a response of lighting up a cigarette, after a meal, on the telephone, with a drink, etc. Clearly the response can be a pleasant one, such as the pleasure that we feel when we hear the voice of a loved one; a picture perhaps or a word that stimulates a warm glow of remembrance of a special event or person – the response that is experienced when a favourite treat is mentioned such as a Black Forest gateau, but then that is my Achilles heel; I wonder what is yours?

These can be termed "conditional responses", the stimulus being associated with a particular event or circumstance, but the important thing for us here is that a response can be controlled if we are able to marry a particular event or stimulus to a desired response or reaction.

A stimulus can be any one of many events, be it taste, feel, colour, hearing or smell. A most useful explanation is the following extract from ***Neuro-Linguistic Programming, Vol 1***:

"Anchoring is in many ways simply the user-oriented version of the stimulus response concept in behaviouristic models. There are however, some major differences between the two. These include:

1)   Anchors do not need to be conditioned over long periods of time in order to be experienced. That kind of conditioning undoubtedly will contribute to the establishment of the anchor, but it is often the initial experience that establishes the anchor most firmly. Anchors then promote the use of single trial learning.

2)   The association between the anchor and the response need not be directly reinforced by any immediate outcome resulting from the association in order to be established. That is, anchors or associations will become established without direct rewards or reinforcement for the association. Reinforcement, like conditioning, will contribute to the establishment of an anchor, but is not required.

3) Internal experience (i.e. cognitive behaviour) is considered to be as significant, behaviourally, as the overt measurable responses; in other words NLP (Neuro-Linguistic Programming) asserts that an internal dialogue, picture or feeling constitutes as much of a response as the salivation of Pavlov's dogs."

Dilts, Grinder, Bandler, Delozier, 1980.

The following script for Nail Biting can be regarded as a generic habit script using anchoring techniques. It will not need great leaps of imagination to see how this format can be used for so many problems by simple substitution of the symptomatic response that is undesirable.

Nail Biting

And now as you relax even deeper, listening to the sound of my voice ....
each word that I speak Here can be a signal for you to go deeper still as
you rest, so comfortable and quiet There. I wonder if you can really be
aware now of how much more comfortable you can become .... as you
begin now to sense in some safe and agreeable way .... a gentle connection
between your mind and your body that has no part to play here .... all that
is required is that you continue to allow those comfortable hypnotic
sensation .... heaviness of arms .... of legs .... comfortably heavy .... to
deepen even more .... as your whole body relaxes .... all tension just
draining away .... and you can turn inward now .... deep inside to where
that part of you that is all-knowing .... creative and perfect .... is ready now
to do its best work for you .... to help you make those changes that you
want to make .... that you can make and will make.

That's good *(client's name)*; now I would like you to allow your
subconscious to take you back in time .... back to a time when you were
really confident in your ability to take control and to be in control .... a
memory of yours .... pleasant and reassuring .... when you really did feel
good .... powerful .... assertive .... and allow that experience to develop and
those good feelings to expand .... and when you are fully experiencing that
event .... I want you to allow your subconscious to lift the pointing finger
of your right hand..... *(ideomotor response)*. If you experience any difficulty
in recalling a memory that is appropriate, then that's fine .... you can allow
your subconscious to create a scene where you are confident and in total
control .... go ahead now ....

*(Watch for responses including skin tone and breathing as well as ideomotor
response.)*

*(Now tell the client that you are going to touch them several times on the shoulder
or arm. Then gently but firmly grasp the shoulder or arm of the client and
continue to maintain the pressure for about 10 to 15 seconds to establish the
anchor.)*

That's good, you are doing this very well .... and now I want you to allow
that scene to fade and your mind to become as before, calm and quiet.
Now I would like you to allow your subconscious mind to show you a
scene .... in the future at one of the next times when you would bite your
nails .... your hands staying where they are now comfortably in your lap

There..... having no part to play Here. .... Allow that scene and that experience to develop and become real .... those feelings to expand and grow .... and you can allow your subconscious to let me know when that is done .... as that pointing finger on your right hand can lift. *(Touch finger.)*

(Watch for responses including skin tone and breathing as well as ideomotor response. Now again grasp firmly the shoulder or arm of the client as exactly before and continue for about 10 to 15 seconds to "fire" the anchor.)

That's fine .... you really are doing this well .... and I wonder now just how you feel about biting your nails .... how you will find it so easy to not do that anymore .... remembering how unpleasant and how bad it made you feel because now you know what you are not going to do .... and how to remind yourself with an irresistible response .... reaching deep into the subconscious of your mind, that you will never ever be able to do that again in that way or at all .... because if you do then you will be doing it on purpose .... and that's a different matter entirely .... it all belongs to you.

Sexual Problems:

Impotence And Inorgasmia

I wonder if you are really aware of those things that are done automatically .... those instinctive things that the body can do for you that need not be learned .... but have been learned in some special way .... like the new-born babe who knows just how to suckle exactly .... and becomes aware of the pleasure that can be from those parts which are sexual .... and in the same way can do those things that you want to do and those things that you want to happen.

Now you have come here because you want to know that you do know how to have those thing happen .... and experience those sensations and pleasures in that special way .... so I would like you now to listen carefully to what I am going to say .... and to what happens to you .... sensations and pleasures that are natural and desirable .... that you can enjoy and continue to enjoy as you begin to know even more than before that you really have known all along how to respond and to never forget that responding.

As you concentrate fully now on my voice and on those sexual sensual parts of you .... where sensations are even now beginning to stir .... I want you to know that there are things that you can think .... images that you can create that can cause those sensations to occur and those physical changes to occur .... thoughts and images that perhaps you would consider inappropriate .... quite indecent perhaps .... but which can stimulate the imagination .... creating scenes for you within the privacy of your own imagination .... erotic and sensual thoughts .... of emotions and sensations .... that will arouse that natural and pleasurable instinctive subconscious reaction to a special wonderful need that is the most natural and beautiful part of our human creation.

You can allow these thoughts to grow..... utilize these feelings that are yours .... fantasies provided for you by that part of you which does know just how to do those things for you .... uninhibited and free of conscious restraint .... and it can enjoy .... as you enjoy allowing those thoughts and images to continue naked and unashamed .... and allowing you now to experience those sensations there .... that touching glow of pleasure .... as you begin to know what a difference that difference can make when they begin to touch .... to caress .... and then to enter in that gentle .... special ....

deep penetrating way .... gently moving to establish a bond and a remembrance that will be there to enjoy as that time comes .... coming together .... and you will come to know that it really is okay to experience in that way .... to give and to receive that special and private gift .... and you can know that when you leave here today that you can experience that softening and that moistening .... that firm feeling that becomes larger and harder to know just how it begins .... as you discover even more than before just how easy it can be to know how that which works for you .... time after time again .... whenever you want or need to .... it all belongs to you.

When you leave here today .... intensely aware that you do know how to do those things .... I would caution you that it can be awkward if you know too well and too often .... you could become excited and aroused all of the time .... just imagine how it would be to be that way .... so full of wanting .... so full of firm desire that it could be so moist .... so hard to contain .... and others may notice too how easy it can be to remember to be ready .... so awkward .... it could be embarrassing.

Taking Responsibility

Metaphor and suggestion for determining what is important:

As you rest quietly there, aware now of that gentle connection between your mind and your perfect inner self .... that part of you that has all those capacities .... knowledge and abilities to solve those problems that are causing you pain .... to create for you so many alternatives that are positive and beneficial to your highest good .... I am reminded of a client of mine who came to see me for help with a problem that he had at work.

Now John had a very good job with an insurance company, and he had a lot of colleagues working with him whom he regarded as friends .... people he would often socialise with and who came to dinner parties at his home .... he had a very good social life indeed.

John was very good at his job and often he would be able to help others with his knowledge and his enthusiasm. Because he worked with people that he regarded as friends, he felt very much that he had a duty to help them in any way that he could. He would sort the problems of his friends because he had confidence in his own abilities and thought that he could do it so much better than they.

He spent a great deal of his time and energy putting the mistakes and omissions of others to rights, ensuring in this way that they would not suffer from their lack of ability and enthusiasm, and lose for the company valuable business. He defended their mistakes and even covered up for them using his own time and energy to visit clients on their behalf to ensure that contracts were finalised.

His friends did very well by him. He worked long hours and took on the stress and the pressure in making absolutely sure that he did all he could to help them. After all, these people were his friends, and true friends will always make sacrifices for those whom they care about.

He failed to take much notice at first of the growing and constant headaches, the tiredness and of the fact that he had become so short-tempered, snapping at his wife and children for no good reason.

He was not too much concerned that the sexual interest in his marriage was now almost non-existent and that his family life seemed to be sliding down a long and slippery slope of constant rows and upsets. His smile had gone, his energy spent and he spent longer and longer hours at the office struggling to complete the immense workload that he had forgotten almost entirely was not his, but that of others.

I wonder if you can imagine his feelings when one day he was called into his superior's office, to be told that a review of personal performance figures had shown that he was producing less business and was now below the average of the rest of the people in his department? He was told that, because of the decline in his performance, the promotion that he had been expecting would not be his, that his performance would be monitored and reviewed on a weekly basis and that he was at risk of losing his position if his performance did not improve.

He went back to his desk, very upset and confused. After all, he knew his job so well and had worked harder and longer than anyone else in the office.

He then discovered that the friend whom he had helped most, whom he had carried and covered for, whose mistakes he had rectified, was the one who had received the promotion that was to be his.

It took a very true and special friend to tell him the truth, and it was with great sadness that he eventually came to the realisation that, in taking on the responsibilities for the lives and the problems of those whom he considered his friends, he had neglected to his own detriment the responsibility that was his, the responsibility for his own health and happiness and for his own wife and children, the responsibility to take for himself the time to ensure the quality of life that was his by right. He took a decision to accept the responsibility that was his, to do that which was beneficial and right for him and for those he loved and cared for.

He had some leave to come and made a decision to take himself and his wife and children away on holiday, and for two glorious weeks devoted all of his energies to putting back that which had been lost. As if by magic, the headaches and the lack-lustre feelings just dissolved away as he involved himself once again with the important and valuable things of life. He relaxed, as you are now so very relaxed, and rediscovered the pleasure of a loving wife and the joys of children .... it did not take long for him to realise the truth, and to recognise that he had become obsessed with taking on the responsibilities of others.

He resolved to take care of the most important elements of his life, his wife and family and himself .... Those who loved him and whom he loved and cared for were where his true responsibilities lay.

When he returned after his holiday, I wonder if you can imagine his feelings to discover that the office was in a state of chaos? His colleagues made it plain to him that they felt that he had let them down by going away and leaving then so much work to do.

It was with great deliberation that he addressed the entire staff that day. He explained to them that he would no longer be prepared to take on their workload and that they would have to accept for themselves the responsibility that was theirs for their own performance. He made plain that he would not interfere in that responsibility but that, if his advice was required, he would be pleased to give the benefit of his experience, but that decisions taken would have to be their own. He spoke of how they would all need to accept their own responsibility for their own life, no more or no less than he was for his; that they were all entitled, as was he, to the rewards for their own efforts and diligence, and not that for which they had been prepared to see him make all that effort, on their behalf.

It didn't take long for the office to fall in line with these new rules and very soon John was back on top where he belonged. He no longer took on any responsibility other than that which was his, and his colleagues soon realised that, with just a bit more effort, they too could do well. They learned to accept the advice that John would give, but also that they needed to ask for that advice and then to accept the responsibility for the decision that needed to be made. Perhaps, too, a lesson was learned that gifts given should be appreciated and treasured, and that kindness improves with the giving.

Experience can be a bitter pill to swallow, as the realisation dawns that even friends will happily allow their responsibilities to be shouldered by another, while they reap the benefit of labour and effort that is not theirs; perhaps you can wonder too that the time given was so greedily taken and then so casually acknowledged.

I know that you will take the time to give to yourself that which you are entitled to, time to care for you, not in an egotistical way, but in a way that will mean that you make those decisions which are right for you and for those whom you love and care for. You accept now, without reservation or pause, the responsibility that can only be yours, and allow others the freedom to choose what is right for them. You wish, for all those around you, the same good feelings of freedom and of confidence in your own abilities and capacities that you enjoy, as you establish yourself as your own person, that person whom you like and respect, a confidant of your own wise inner advisor as you allow that wonderful feeling of oneness with yourself to expand and cocoon you now with its soothing light of beneficial calm and positivity. Now you are your own person .... are you not?

(Await response and go to trance termination).

Pleasure Returned

Metaphor and suggestion for premature ejaculation.

I wonder if you have ever had that pleasure of looking around a beautiful garden .... and wonder just how you can best appreciate the wonders that are there .... the carefully planted borders .... the colours and the variety of plants all creating a harmony, and then a complementary variance .... blooms each in their time throughout the whole of the four seasons .... You can see those who will look at all that is there .... darting from this plant to that shrub, so full of wonder that they really cannot decide which to look at .... which to savour and appreciate first .... there is so much to enjoy .... so much to savour .... the shouts of joyous discovery .... look at this .... look at that .... isn't it lovely .... beautiful .... then to rush on to the next .... so much beauty .... so much colour .... confusing and confounding .... the wanting to see it all .... Now .... enjoy it all .... Now .... miss nothing .... have it all .... so they rush without giving time to express the real appreciation in a controlled and considered manner.

There are those who cultivate these delights .... tilling the soil and ensuring that what is offered is of ultimate beauty .... ensuring that the colour and the variety is ever there .... waiting for that time when the garden is open .... the public allowed in .... its pleasures to be enjoyed .... Those who take the time .... who make available to us the pleasures that will be provided with love and with gentle care .... can watch as those who would enjoy, take their pleasure .... those who take more time .... relaxing and experiencing as they look at each and every petal .... every leaf .... every branch .... so many varieties .... savouring the essence of natural joy in those things which are as nature intended .... will also take the time to seek out the gardener .... the provider of all of this pleasure .... this sensual delight .... and extend to that person who has given so much of themselves .... the thanks and appreciation which are also to be enjoyed .... then giving and receiving so much more as that interest .... that gentle consideration is rewarded with personal attention and direction to the hidden delights .... the subtle pleasures .... extending the time of pleasure with pleasurable anticipation .... taking the time now to enjoy each step .... each movement, each new experience..... and learning more of that gardener's pleasure in what is provided there .... pausing to allow time to explore even more than before those areas of pleasure that are hidden from those who rush by .... even trampled and crushed underfoot .... murmurings of pleasure .... appreciation of that beauty and that care .... reverence and respect ....

allowing the beauty to embrace and enfold .... that takes them into another quiet and tranquil experience away from the hurry and scurry of those who will see only what is there for them .... too excited .... too uncontrolled to share .... and it can be so satisfying knowing that when all is done .... all is appreciated and that appreciation expressed .... that pleasure returned and shared .... that it really is okay to let go in that way .... letting that feeling grow, allowing those emotions to explode in a couplet of delight .... then to tarry a while .... knowing that they really can .... and can return again and again .... and each time more is discovered .... the gardener becomes a trusted and beloved companion .... each visit a sharing experience as knowledge grows and each of those pleasures can become something that happens time after time as your subconscious mind finds new and more exciting .... pleasurable ways for you .... with an understanding of those things which are there all of the time .... hidden within the realms of your higher mind .... now shown in a wonderful clarity to you as you learn even more about those things that are done for you in that way .... automatically.

So now you can relax deeper now .... in communion with that special and all-knowing part of your perfect mind .... that does know how .... and then the next time that you enter into that garden .... perhaps to plant the seeds .... that sown with love will blossom and bloom .... I am sure that you will too take the time to prepare the richness of the soil and give appropriate consideration for the miracle that is yours to enjoy .... and I know too that you will remember to recognize that time when the garden is in bloom and the blossoms open .... the soil moist and receptive .... as the bees know that time, to then allow that conclusion .... that pollination .... that climax to come .... it's completely up to you to enjoy yourself .... or to enjoy yourself giving enjoyment and pleasure .... in return as you take your time .... to pause .... to allow that your love .... your appreciation be appreciated too .... and you will .... will you not?

Pain Management:

Switches For Pain

Now, before you wake up completely, I would like you to just close your eyes again and allow that drifting down again, entering again that place of calm relaxation, because there was a young boy on TV not long ago, who had learned to control all of his pain. He described the steps that he went down in his mind, one at a time down those steps, until he found this hall at the bottom, like a long tunnel, and all along this tunnel on both side were many different switches and switchboxes, all clearly labelled. One for the right hand, one for the left, one for each leg, a switch for every part of the body, and he could see clearly the wires that carried the sensations from one place to another, all going through those switches.

All he needed to do here was to reach up in his mind and turn off the switches that he wanted to, and then he could feel nothing at all, no sensation could get through from there, because he had turned off the appropriate switches there.

He used his mind's abilities differently from the man who simply made his body numb. He didn't know how he did it exactly. All he knew was, he relaxed and disconnected from the rest, moved his mind away from his body, moved it outside somewhere else, where he could watch and listen, but drift off somewhere else entirely. It really doesn't matter how you tell your subconscious what to do, or how your unconscious does it for you. The only thing of importance is that you know you can lose sensations as easily as closing your eyes, and drifting down within where something unknown happens that allows you to disconnect, that allows that numbness to occur, and then a drifting back upwards now, towards the surface, and slowly opening the eyes as wakeful awareness returns with a comfortable continuation of that feeling of safe, secure relaxation and an ability to forget an arm, or anything at all, with no need to pay attention to things that are just fine, that somebody else can take care of for a while, while you drift in your mind and then return when it is time to enjoy that comfortable drifting upwards where the eyes open and wakeful awareness returns completely .... NOW.

The Dentist

Now as you sit comfortably there with your eyes closed .... comfortable and aware that you are here because you want to learn to use your own subconscious abilities to help you to eliminate that discomfort you experience .... that anxiety .... when you visit your dentist. And so .... as you begin to relax and to drift down into trance .... deeper now .... into a deep trance state .... I want you to take your time .... not go too quickly .... yet .... because there are some things that you need to first understand .... so please listen carefully now.

First you need to understand that you already have the ability to lose an arm .... or a hand .... to become totally unaware of just where that arm is positioned .... or the fingers .... and you do have an ability to be unconcerned about exactly where that ear or thumb went .... or that hand .... that leg .... or your entire body .... which may seem to require too much effort to pay attention to at times. Because you do have an ability .... a subconscious ability you can learn to use .... an ability to turn off the sensation in an arm .... a leg .... or even your face .... your jaw .... your gum .... in fact any place.

And once you discover how it feels to feel nothing at all .... whenever you want or need that to occur .... then you can create a comfortable, numb feeling any time .... anywhere that is useful for you.

And I don't know if your unconscious mind can allow you to discover that numb feeling in the right hand .... or a finger of the left hand first .... a tiny area of numbness .... a comfortable tickly feeling .... a heavy .... enveloping numbness .... that seems to spread within time .... over the back of the hand .... covering that hand .... or any part of you that you direct your attention to .... it just fades away .... but you don't know how it feels to feel that something that is not there .... so I would like you to just reach over to that numb, comfortable area .... that numb, comfortable hand .... now .... touch it .... and feel that touching .... as you begin to pinch yourself there .... a sensation that you may be aware of at first .... but as you continue to pinch yourself .... something special happens here .... you begin to experience and discover that there are times when you feel nothing at all there .... that sensation just seems to fade away .... as you learn how to allow your subconscious mind to do that for you .... to turn off those sensations .... and as that ability grows and you become more aware .... that you really do know how .... to really turn off that part .... really know how to switch off those sensations and allow that pain and discomfort to just disappear from that hand .... or from anywhere .... your other hand can return to its resting position .... and you can drift up now towards the surface of wakeful awareness .... so go ahead now as you relax .... and discover how to let go .... and to re-experience that numbness more and more clearly .... and so you can drift up .... and then back down, as you learn even more about your own ability .... in your own time .... in your own way .... you can practise this self-learning .... this ability to do that for you at any time .... at any place.

(Give the client time to practise this technique a few times, and then continue.....)

Now (*client's name*), with your eyes closed .... you can relax more deeply than before .... aware of that new learning .... that new ability to switch off that discomfort .... You can visualize now as vividly as you can .... see yourself at your next visit to your dentist .... please notice now how calm you are feeling as you check in at the desk .... in plenty of time for your appointment.

You now sit in the waiting area .... feeling calm and unconcerned .... confident in your ability to control those sensations .... you smile at others who are waiting with you .... pleased to be able to allow your own calm and confident manner to soothe the minds of others .... as they wait to be called.

As you wait there, you practise again your ability to turn off that sensation there .... and experience now that numbness .... as the sensation in your gums just fades .... that numbness spreading .... just as if you had been given a shot of local anaesthetic .... that woolly, thick feeling of no feeling at all .... and you relax experiencing a total inner calm.

When your turn comes to be called for your appointment .... you take a long deep breath .... and as you expel all the air from your lungs .... you breathe out anxiety .... fear .... and then breathe in calm .... confidence .... tranquillity.

As you sit in the dentist's chair .... you will experience a comfortable sensation as calm fills your mind .... as you relax .... concentrating now on that switch that will allow you to experience that sensation of no sensation .... as your dentist gently and carefully begins the work that is needed to be done.

If he needs to give you anaesthesia, you will be calm and comfortable .... but I really do not want you to giggle when you experience that tickle ....

and may I mention too that I wouldn't want you to drift off too deeply into a trance too quickly as the sound of the drill and the gentle soothing vibrations relax you and calm you .... you will be pleasurably surprised at how calm and relaxed you will become as your dentist .... appreciating your necessary co-operation .... completes his work easily .... skillfully .... you will enjoy being that person who relaxes in that chair and allows your subconscious to utilize that special ability that you have learned .... looking forward to your regular check-ups .... no longer bothered or concerned as you now take control of that fear .... and unlearn that fear .... seeing it now for exactly what it was .... no longer imagining in that way that tells you that there are things to fear here .... as your subconscious mind takes care of you .... takes care of those thoughts those feelings automatically .... aware that you can trust you to be okay, with no need to pay attention to things that are just fine .... things that somebody else can just take care of .... and it doesn't really matter exactly how you tell your subconscious mind what to do or how your subconscious mind does it for you .... the only thing of importance is that you know that you can lose those sensations .... those discomforts .... just as easily as closing your eyes .... while you drift in your mind and then return when it is time .... back to wakeful awareness .... quite completely now.

Therapy Strategies:

Six-Step Reframe

Basic Steps:

1. Identify the habit or compulsive pattern of behaviour [X] to be changed.

2. Establish communication with that part that has been responsible for [X].

3. Suggest that behaviour [X] be separated from the positive intervention of the part responsible for [X]: in other words, [X] has had pay-offs or benefits for the client.

4. Suggest that the client generate new behaviours that provide the needed pay-offs.

5. Do an "ecological check". Are the alternative patterns of behaviour acceptable to all parts of the person ?

6. Future pace. Check out the alternative patterns of behaviour within relevant future contexts.

Technique:

Take a few deep breaths now, and make yourself comfortable, relaxing deeper with each easy breath that you take, and take a few moments to concentrate on that *(insert habit or behaviour)* that you wish to change, but something is stopping you.

Now that you know that changing this habit is important to you, I would like you to know that I have so often found that the part which is preventing you from making the change you want to make is an unconscious part of you.

If that is the case here, I would like to ask that part of you to now make itself known, in some safe way, to your unconscious mind. Please take a few moments of time to go into your own inner mind – wherever you have to go – and become aware of the part of you which, in the past, has been responsible for *(insert habit or behaviour)*.

Now I don't know exactly how you will experience that part of you which has been responsible for *(insert habit or behaviour)* .... It may be a familiar type of experience, or a unique one .... It may be something you see in your mind's eye: it can be any visual image at all .... For example, you may see a face or an object, or the experience of that inner part of you may be auditory .... such as a voice – perhaps your own, or someone else's – or some other sound .... Your experience of that part of you may be a feeling of some kind.

Please go into your own inner mind now .... With respect I ask that part of you to allow itself to be experienced in some kind of safe comfortable way by your consciousness .... If you do not become aware of any particular experience which can be identified as an awareness that is responsible, ... then that is fine, ... please proceed with the understanding that your subconscious may not be just comfortable with your experiencing what I have suggested, and that's all right .... If you are experiencing that part of you which is responsible for *(insert habit or behaviour)*, I would like now to thank that part for communicating, and to suggest that you might also wish to thank that part.

I want now to let the part of you responsible for *(insert habit or behaviour)* in the past know that it has my respect .... That part is obviously very powerful, because even though you have wanted to make this change in the past, you haven't been able to do so. Therefore I understand that this part of you responsible for your problem will change it only when it is ready to do so.

I would now like to suggest to you that, in some kind of way, *(insert habit or behaviour)* has had benefits or pay-offs for you in the past, that you have in some way gained an advantage .... I understand that the actual experience or behaviour of that part has caused negative or unhealthy consequences for you, but I am suggesting that you now reframe your understanding of it to realise that the intention of that part of you has been to help you or benefit you. Now take a few moments of time to go into your own inner mind and become aware of what the pay-offs or benefits of *(insert habit or behaviour)* have been for you.

Has *(insert habit or behaviour)* helped get something that some part of you has desired *(give example of possible pay-off)*. .... Has it helped you avoid something that would be uncomfortable or painful *(possible example)*? .... I am asking you again to assume that *(insert behaviour or habit)* has continued up to now because it has helped you or benefited you in some way. So *(client's name)*, please become aware, if it is safe and comfortable enough to have this awareness, of how *(insert habit or behaviour)* has helped you.

Now, keeping the pay-off or pay-offs in mind, ... I would like to suggest that available to you are alternative patterns of behaviour, ... of experiencing, ... or perception, that can provide whatever benefits or pay-offs *[insert behaviour or habit]* you had in the past. However, these new patterns of behaviour would be healthier and perhaps even more satisfying to you. .... Now take some moments of time and go into your mind again.

Tap into the creative resources of your mind and allow it to generate for you alternative patterns of behaviour that you can substitute for *(insert habit or behaviour)*, that will give you the same pay-offs as *(insert habit or behaviour)*, but be healthier for you.

Now that you have constructed alternative patterns of behaviour, the next step is to check with that part of you that was responsible for *(insert habit or behaviour)*, as well as all the other parts of you, that they will be comfortable and satisfied with the new alternatives.

Would you go into your mind again and make sure that all the new alternatives seem all right, ... sound all right .... and feel all right to that part of you that was responsible for *(insert habit or behaviour)*, and to all parts of you.

If you receive a "no" signal, or in any way experience incongruence from any part of you - for example irritability or increase in tension - in response to your new alternative or alternatives, then it is necessary that you return to a prior step of reframing. You may need to go back and allow your creative part to generate a new alternative or alternatives. Or you may have to go back even further to identify and take into account some benefit or pay-off that you were not aware of before. If your new alternatives are okay, then I would like you to go back into your inner mind to take part in an exercise called "future pacing".

Please now go into your inner mind again and imagine yourself in the future on occasions when you would have, in the past, indulged in *(insert habit or behaviour)*. Imagine yourself in these future contexts with the ability to use these new alternative patterns of behaviour that you have just become aware of.

Imagine yourself in these future contexts with these alternative patterns. If you experience significant difficulty, it may be necessary for you to generate more suitable alternatives. When you have completed generating for yourself suitable alternatives which are beneficial and healthy, and have imagined successfully future contexts with alternative patterns of behaviour, then you have completed the process of reframing. I would suggest now that you thank your subconscious mind for communicating in that way, and I would like to express my appreciation for the healthy work that you have just completed and extend my thanks for the valuable communication.

Use suggestion for amnesia. Go to trance termination and do not discuss session content with client before he/she leaves.

Original concept : Bandler/Grinder, *Reframing,* **1982**

Parts Therapy

Generic

1. Explain the concept to the client before inducing hypnosis. The procedure is not dependent upon this explanation, but will serve to allay any problems alluding to "Multiple Personality"

2. Induce hypnosis using your choice of induction and deepener.

3. Tell the client:
   "You can speak to me now but you will not wake. .... I am now going to speak directly to your subconscious mind .... and I want to speak specifically to that part which is responsible for *(detail problem)* .... Are you the part of *(client's name)* that is responsible for this problem *(detail problem)*? .... Please answer 'yes' or 'no'."

4. Having received a positive response, thank the part for coming forward:
   "Thank you for coming forward today and speaking with me .... please tell me your name .... are you male or female?"

5. Ask how old the whole person was when the part first appeared .... encourage dissociation by proper use of pronouns.
   "How old was *(client's name)* when you first appeared?" *(Note: The ego state is usually "young", so address it in simple language).*

6. "Tell me *(name of part)* what was happening to *(client's name)* that caused you to first appear?" *(Elicit elaboration of those events).*

7. Now attempt to define the part's goal:
   "So, you appeared in order to *(punish, comfort, etc.)* .... Is that true?"

8. Comment on the value of the goal and its appropriateness. Redefine it in positive terms.

9. Offer an alternative and more appropriate method of obtaining these goals; .... ask for the part's co-operation in trying out these new methods for just one week to see how they work out.

10. Thank the part for its co-operation and assure it that you will check progress with it at the next session:
    "Thank you for coming forward to speak to me today, and for the co-operation that you have shown. I would like to ask if there is any other part that objects to this arrangement? *(Provided there is a negative response:)* You may return now from where you came .... I will speak with you at our next session."

11. Trance termination:
    "When I complete a count of three, the whole person that is *(client's name)* will open his/her eyes and return to fully-awake awareness .... remembering everything of this session that can be handled comfortably."

12. Use distraction to discourage rationalization of the session content; .... terminate session as quickly as is respectfully possible.

Strategy For Past-Life Recall
(P.L.R.)

Before embarking on a past-life recall, I explain carefully to the client the powers of the imagination and the nature of memory. It is important that the client is aware of the possibility that memories recalled may be simply those of watching a film or reading a book, or even just an imagined event. The subconscious memory does not differentiate and will accept all memory as actuality. What the client chooses to accept as truth must be left entirely to them. Whether or not you, the therapist, accept or deny the truth of the events occurring is of no consequence).

Carry out a lengthy induction:

Deepening with imagery:

"Now I would like you to imagine yourself in a place that will provide for you feelings of peace and comfort .... security .... tranquillity .... It may be winter, summer, ... spring or autumn .... there may be trees .... mountains .... water .... lush green meadows .... or perhaps a beach with the waves rolling in from the ocean .... whichever place you choose will have great peace and harmony, and you feel totally safe and secure here .... and as you become more and more involved with this place that you have chosen, you can relax even deeper than before .... relaxing .... releasing .... just letting go completely.

This is your own private and secret place, and you are aware that this place is your own haven deep inside where only peace and harmony abide .... and you can go so much deeper now .... turning inward to your innermost self .... where all knowledge and all memories are kept safe for you .... some easily accessible .... others hidden deep where they can not be so easily recalled .... but they are there .... each and every one .... never forgotten from so far back in this life and a time when this life was not yet begun .... memories that have shaped and moulded your unique and special personality .... and as you go deep inside now .... you can begin to experience a gentle connection with that special part of you which holds those memories that you now wish to explore and to re- experience .... that part now makes itself known to you in some special and safe way that you can recognize easily .... Tell me *(client's name)*, do you have any special or strange feelings or sensations? *(Wait for response)* .... *(When your client reports any strange or unusual sensation, sound or image, continue).*

Okay, that's good .... now let that feeling or experience grow stronger as you go deeper inside to connect more fully with that part of you. .... Now I am going to speak directly to your subconscious mind, and I am going to ask your subconscious for permission to conduct a past-life recall .... I want your subconscious to give me the answer .... please do not do anything at all .... just continue to enjoy the peace and comfort of this place that you have chosen.

(The use of ideomotor response can be utilized at this juncture .... see script on page 21.)

I am now going to touch your forehead and ask the question. My words go directly into your subconscious and the answer, either 'yes' or 'no', will come directly from that part of you. Please do not involve yourself at all as your subconscious mind provides the answer to my question. *(Touch centre of forehead with finger.)*

Am I speaking to that part of *(client's name)* which is able to give me permission to conduct a past-life recall .... answer 'yes' or 'no' .... *(Wait for response. If answer is 'yes' you can proceed).* Thank you, subconscious mind, for communicating with me .... I have been asked by *(client's name)* to help him/her to go back to that time, before this life, to a previous existence .... Do I have your permission to do this and your help in this? Answer 'yes' or 'no'.

(Await response. If response is 'yes', then continue).

Thank you, subconscious mind .... I know that you are there to ensure that all that is revealed will be done in a manner that is safe and beneficial for *(client's name)*.

(Remove finger from forehead).

Now *(client's name)*, we can proceed but first, for your protection, I want you now to see around you forming a white light .... a warm and comforting glow that will surround you and envelop you in its protective aura .... a safe, protective cocoon that will remain with you throughout the coming experience and beyond. Know now that I am with you at all times and that at any time .... if I touch you on the shoulder like this *(touch shoulder with a firm but gentle pressure)* .... you can then immediately safely return to this time and this place .... here .... now .... to safety and peace, and nothing can harm you or disturb you at all.

Now I am going to count to three and then snap my fingers .... and you will find yourself with me in a long corridor that stretches back through time .... right back through to the beginning of this life. You will see that there are many doors on either side of the corridor, and behind each of these doors are stored memories of this life .... some good, some bad and then some that your subconscious mind has kept from you .... as you walk along the corridor, as you pass each of these doors, you will be aware of feelings and emotions .... images .... sounds and experiences that emanate from within each of those rooms behind each of those doors. It may be that behind one of these doors is a memory that has been causing you pain in this life .... a memory of an event that needs to be addressed here and now .... your subconscious mind will guide you here and, should there be a particular door which merits your attention, you will be drawn to that door .... and you will know that, before we proceed further, that door must be opened and you must deal with what lies within that room beyond.

So go ahead now .... walk along that corridor, past each of those doors .... ahead of you at the other end of the corridor you can see in the distance a door .... so much heavier .... so much more imposing than all of those along the sides .... this is the door through which you passed into this life from beyond .... and it is this door that you must now go through to see what was before, and it awaits you now .... you have the key and it will open for you .... but you must pass by all of the other doors of this life before you can pass through this one. Go ahead now .... take your time .... if there is a door that beckons you before you reach that special door, then that is okay, and we can pause to deal with whatever needs to be done .... you can speak to me clearly now as we go ahead .... but you cannot wake .... just tell me when you are at the door to that life before .... or a door that needs to be opened here before we go on .... I am with you at all times.

(Events as they occur will determine progress. It may well be the case that the client will feel drawn to a door on this side of the veil. Here you should proceed, allowing him/her to enter that room and deal with the content which may be the cause of some problems in this life. Proceed down the corridor when the client feels able to leave that room .... into the corridor and then firmly close the door on the memory accessed, having dealt with it in an appropriate and beneficial way. You, as the therapist, must use your best judgment).

Now as you stand before that door that all those years ago you passed through to enter into this life, are you now certain that you wish to open that door and step through to whatever lies beyond?

(Await response)

Okay, that's fine, I want you now to see the key to that door in the lock .... reach out now and turn that key .... feel it turn easily .... now push open that door. Now I will count to three and on the count of three you will find yourself in a time before this time .... this life .... in a place where you have been in another time .... where you have lived before. One .... Two .... Three. .... Where are you now? Are you inside a building or outside? How old are you? .... What is your name? ....

(The questions that you ask will of necessity be in accordance with the natural progression of the client's experience. The main points at this stage are to ascertain details of age, sex, nationality and profession. Questions as to family and friends, etc. .... to determine the period in which this life was lived. I remember many years ago being advised to allow my own subconscious to help me and in this I will pass on that good advice. I personally record the sessions in order that facts which arise can be checked by the client if that is his/her wish)

(At the end of every life, there is a death, and this is a matter which can be important to the client's experience. Obviously, there can be violence, sometimes horrific events, but you have assured your client that he/she is beyond harm. Remember to use the name that is given in the life recalled when speaking to your client.)

Now (*client's name*), in a moment I am going to count from one to three and then I will snap my fingers .... you will then find yourself at that time at that place just before you pass into spirit. **"Snap"**! Please tell me where you are and what is happening to you. *(Here you will be exploring the circumstances of death - it could be sickness, violence or just old age .... the client may have died alone or with others around .... yours are the questions that will bring out the facts).*

Now, when I snap my fingers you will leave this life, passing into spirit. **"Snap!"**

Now let's go to your funeral: .... who is there? .... what does it say on your memorial?, etc. etc ....

When I snap my fingers again, I want you to find yourself in that place where all souls go between lives .... **"Snap!"** .... Describe to me now this place where you are .... are there any people in this life that you have recalled that are there with you now? Are there any people there, who will be with you in your next life, the life that you have been living before you went back to that life before?

What was the purpose of the life that you have just recalled? .... Were you successful in that life, ... achieving that purpose?

Now, as I count from one to five, I want you to find your way back to that door through which you came to this life recalled .... now go through that door into the corridor and then firmly close that door behind you and turn the key. *(Count slowly from one to five).*

Now I want you to go back to that place of comfort and safety where you were before we began the recall .... now relax and enjoy the peace and the calm tranquillity of this place .... notice now that the white light that enveloped you .... is still with you .... all around you .... that protective aura .... and as you relax deeper now .... that white light begins to enter into your body to be absorbed .... to become part of you, and you can feel its positive force .... its comforting energy as it circulates within your body now .... relaxing you .... calming you .... you feel an emotional calm that cancels out any unpleasant feelings and emotions that you may have had, and you feel more relaxed and comfortable than you have ever felt before.

In a few moments, you will be able to return to full conscious awareness. You will remember everything that is safe and beneficial for you to remember about your previous life recalled, your experience will strengthen you and help you to better understand those things in life which will remain forever unclear, and you will be aware of feelings of peace and calm .... a gentle acceptance of what is to be allows you to continue now, free of anxiety about what will be, as that new understanding deep within your subconscious is utilized to your highest benefit.

Trance termination.

(For the benefit of those like Tony Powell Dp Hp MIAH, who is unable to snap his fingers, the tapping of the desk with a suitable object will serve just as well.)

Releasing Negative Emotions

As you go deeper now .... you can be aware that negative emotions never change anything .... they are simply a waste of energy and a lost opportunity to generate beneficial emotions .... positive thoughts and feelings that will help you.

Negative emotions are hurtful .... they hurt you .... they actually damage and injure you.

When you experience .... anger .... frustration .... guilt .... or jealousy .... this is because you are not getting something that you desire. Agree with yourself right now to stop wanting things that you know you cannot have .... as you do this for yourself .... immediately you will become happier and more content with what you do have.

Agree now to change the way that you think about things .... longing for things you cannot have is ignoring and wasting the benefits and happiness that are to be enjoyed with what you do have. You now decide to enjoy and be happy with what you do have.

If you are harbouring now any negative thoughts and feelings towards others .... they only do you harm .... they actually do cause you harm and pain. Negative thoughts and negative feelings only hold you there in the past .... they prevent you from moving forward .... making progress .... making the most of your life.

If you are harbouring any negative emotions .... anger .... frustration .... or jealousy .... release these feelings .... these negative emotions now .... let them go and forever free yourself from what has been and now is no more.

If you have sadness .... perhaps for something or someone that you have lost .... grieve now for what you have lost .... or for what you never had and release that longing .... that craving .... just let it go.

If you have any guilt for something that you did .... or omitted to do .... forgive yourself .... do it now .... just let it go. You have always done your best in any situation .... you did what was right for you at the time .... or you did what you did because it was all you could do. Just release all guilt right now .... release it whole-heartedly .... just let it go.

You have always done your best .... and nobody can expect that you do more .... so accept that you are the best that you can be and let those negative feelings of inadequacy .... failure .... and guilt go.... just let them go now ....

If you have bad feelings .... feelings of betrayal .... of jealousy .... revenge .... you recognize now with clarity and understanding .... that those feelings do not benefit you in any way .... they harm you .... they hurt you and prevent you concentrating your best efforts on enjoying what you have: .... love .... and warmth .... friendship .... and so much more .... and you release those feelings .... those negative harmful emotions .... just let them go .... they have no place in your life.

When you leave here today, your subconscious will help you with new learnings and positive thoughts and emotions .... It will remind you in a very powerful manner whenever you experience a negative thought .... such as fear .... disgust .... anger .... guilt .... hatred .... jealousy .... that you have a choice .... you can control your thoughts .... control your feelings .... and decide to have only good thoughts and positive emotions .... you choose now to have only good and positive thoughts and feelings. In future you will be aware when you experience a negative thought or emotion .... and you will immediately turn it into a positive thought or emotion .... that helps you to move forward .... enjoy your life and what you do have .... love .... compassion .... understanding .... forgiveness and acceptance of what is to be.

Now you can choose to release all of those negative thoughts .... negative feelings .... right now .... immediately .... or you can choose to do this for yourself in one hour from now .... or just before you go to bed.

Now I would prefer that you release each and every negative thought and feeling right now .... but it is up to you to choose a time .... today .... which is the right time for you .... accepting that your subconscious knows what to do for you .... thinking .... without awareness .... thoughts that are beneficial and appropriate and not needing to know how it will do that for you.

Now as you go deeper .... turning inward .... becoming one with your own inner mind .... that part of you that has perfect knowledge and understanding .... I would like you to allow that part of you to do its best work for you as you present to your inner self all of those negative thoughts, feelings and emotions that have in the past hurt you .... and enjoy the warm comfortable positive feeling that embraces you now as those negatives are dealt with in a most appropriate manner .... released ....

disposed of to be replaced with positive beneficial thoughts .... feelings .... and emotions.

Present to your subconscious now .... each of those negative emotions that you have experienced .... present each seven times .... and experience now the strength and the comfort as each negative emotion is transformed .... easily .... quickly .... and without effort. When you have finished this task and you are completely satisfied that all the work that needs to be done for your benefit .... has been completed .... then you can allow yourself to drift upwards .... towards the surface of awareness .... bringing with you feelings of balance .... positivity .... confidence .... and good feelings about your own self worth as a special and unique person .... allowing your eyes to open feeling refreshed .... feeling wonderful.

Sleep & Dream

The unconscious mind is interesting to observe as you drift down into that trance .... where those unconscious thoughts and images and ideas .... flash through the mind like schools of fish darting through a clear blue sea .... startling as they suddenly appear .... their strange shapes and forms .... and then disappear to be replaced by others .... beautiful .... strange .... wonderful.

Some thoughts and images are of the past .... about the present .... or about the future .... and perhaps you will know how pleasant it can seem to see that what is to come can be good .... pleasant .... and beneficial .... or perhaps that all will be sad .... unpleasant .... and detrimental .... like frightened fortune-tellers of days gone by .... predicting the end of the world .... seeing the gloom and misfortune to come in the manner in which tea leaves are left behind in a cup when all else has been enjoyed .... All they can see is what is bad.

When you look at your hands .... I wonder if what you see there is the future .... or is it the past that you see there .... or even the present? .... And is what you see there good or bad .... or just what must be there at present? .... Real fingers .... real thumbs .... and do the fingers point to the past or to what will be .... who can tell? .... And what do you make of the horoscopes in the daily papers and how they will suggest that wealth .... health .... and happiness are just around the corner .... that every cloud has a silver lining .... while the prophets of doom are abroad with their placards and slogans .... announcing the end of mankind and the wrath of heaven?

Those who are paid .... are paid attention to and have a different point of view .... but at least their messages are easy to see .... not hidden away to pop out to remind us of how bad .... how awful things could be .... telling us to beware of this, or afraid of that .... reminding us to be concerned at something that could happen .... something awful or even terrible .... and I wonder if you really do see yourself falling each time you walk down those stairs .... or trapping fingers each time that you close a door .... and how often does that terrible predicted thing occur, and how often did it **not** occur, time after time after time.

Please consider now those birds who, as soon as they are born, ... are afraid .... They don't have to learn to fear the shape of a hawk that soars above .... nature does that for them to protect them .... and on some large buildings with lots of glass .... that shape of the hawk is pasted on the glass windows to stop the birds from flying into them and harming themselves.

The shape scares them away and that cannot be unlearned. You know that you will not fall off the edge of the world if you sail out to sea .... you know that tomatoes are not poisonous .... and that toads will not give you warts .... and just believing that you can fly .... will not make it so .... even though it can be fun to watch Superman or Peter Pan .... like anything can be fun or not .... and any knot can be untied .... as your unconscious mind finds its own way to unlearn for you and see things in a different light .... a warm .... positive .... comfortable light that allows things to change .... feelings to change .... to rearrange those thoughts and images .... allowing the mind to foresee that change in the future and to enjoy noticing that change occur.

And now as you relax in that very special way .... your unconscious mind for your benefit makes itself open to all the suggestions that I might make here .... which are all for your benefit .... and allow those suggestions to imprint deep in your inner mind .... firmly fixed .... embedded so that they remain with you long after you leave here today .... helping you to learn new ways to make those changes that you want to make for your own sake.

And so for now .... you can enjoy that feeling of deep and special relaxation .... aware of those inner forces empowering you .... enabling you to grow stronger .... fitter .... more confident in your own special abilities and capacities to do those things which are right for you .... to concentrate your mind on those things which are positive and rewarding.

You become aware of your special qualities .... recognize your own true worth .... your thoughts from this moment are directed outwards from yourself to what you sense around you .... You become more relaxed .... steadier .... more settled .... mentally and physically.

At the end of each day you will be pleasantly tired .... remaining calm and confident in your new-found learnings about yourself .... and you will then settle down in your bed as your unconscious mind reminds you that it really is okay to be okay and to let go now .... and to give yourself permission to sleep a deep and restful sleep .... readying you for the day to come .... a day when you will feel stronger and feel better .... and each day you will become stronger and fitter .... more alive .... more confident in your ability to look after you in a way that your subconscious will find easy .... automatic to do for you.

I will give you an anchor now .... you can know that your subconscious mind will be there to protect and guide you through the hours of the night .... letting you know that it is okay .... and to let you know that should your attention be required .... should a child call out for you .... that you are instantly awake and aware .... then you relax again and resume that restful deep slumber when all is well .... and all is well.

And now as you continue to relax .... each breath soothing you .... I wonder how much attention you have paid to the different thoughts floating through your mind .... your mind can be so active as it relaxes .... and then you can realise how difficult it is to remember what I was saying exactly seven minutes ago .... or what I was talking about nine minutes ago .... or what you were thinking about .... four minutes ago .... but doesn't it seem like too much effort to bother trying to remember? .... It takes more effort than it's worth .... and so will you remember to just relax comfortably .... when it really is too much work .... too much effort to bother at all.

And so for now you can take some time .... for yourself to go over it all and review all that you have experienced there while your body rests so comfortably here .... so go ahead now .... take a short time that can seem to be a long time .... and you can let me know when you have done all that is needed .... returning to the surface of wakeful awareness .... bringing with you that new feeling of balance and harmony .... feeling restful and relaxed .... confident and assured .... feeling absolutely wonderful .... as you appreciate what an eye-opening experience it has been.

The Final Good-Bye

For use with those clients who have lost someone and did not have the opportunity to say good-bye and to say those things that needed to be said.

Contra-indications: those who will not accept the concept of continuance of spiritual being.

(Induce hypnosis and use "The Garden" deepener)

In this beautiful and serene place where you are so comfortable and relaxed .... where peace and harmony are so natural .... you can be aware that it can be so easy to relax even deeper now as you listen to the sound of my voice .... each word a signal for you to go deeper and deeper still into profound relaxation of mind and body .... and did you know that just as you have eyes that see the world around you .... you also have an eye deep within that we call the mind's eye? .... And, just like your physical eyes, this eye has an eyelid that can close down .... as you relax, it will close down shutting out those stray thoughts and images that are not appropriate here .... and it is closing now .... closing .... closing .... and all that is there now is calm tranquillity .... feelings of peace and of capability .... of beneficial possibility.

And as you relax ever deeper you can be aware that, although you are alone in this beautiful place .... many before you have come here to enjoy and benefit from the positive healing vibrations that abound here .... and I would like you to know that you have been so very fortunate to have known that special person who has so quickly been taken from you .... fortunate that you have been able to hold such wonderful memories that have been for you so powerful .... so influential.

In this special place .... you can enjoy today a very rare and special privilege .... for here .... there in that garden of peace .... all must pass in spirit as they travel to that place beyond the gate in the wall at the bottom of the garden .... the gate that you can see now through the screen of trees .... overgrown with ivy and honeysuckle .... a gate through which you cannot pass .... yet .... for you have much to do here .... your life to live.

You can be aware of the sounds of gentle laughter .... of music and of an aura of peace that you have not yet experienced .... this is coming from beyond the gate .... in that place where all departed spirits dwell between lives .... where even now there are those who have gone before who wait for you .... watching you and lending to you the strength that they can give to you in spirit.

You are now standing before that gate .... carved and ornate, it stands firmly bolted for you are not ready to enter .... but just for a time you have the gift now of asking someone within to pass through that gate into the garden here .... and for a time you can speak with that person .... ask what you need to ask and know that the answers will be given with truth and wisdom that is no longer constrained and influenced by the matters of this world. Those beyond that gate have passed through the veil that keeps from the living the truths and the wisdom, and they now are unfettered by those earthly constraints .... All you need to do is to call the name of that person .... and they will come through that gate to speak with you. Because that person is in spirit and formless, I don't know how they will make themselves known to you .... you may see them as you know that person .... or perhaps you will experience a feeling .... an emotion that lets you know that they are there .... but you will know that that person is there .... in some safe, pleasant way and for a time you can speak with that person .... say all of those things that you want to say .... ask all that you need to ask .... and know that here there is only love.

It is different this time .... for you know that soon, very soon, he/she must return beyond the gate .... there to wait for you .... but this time you can be sure that all that needs to be said can be said and that the peace you seek can be real .... so that you can release him/her and then continue with the life that you have .... make the choices that you can make .... positive and beneficial .... moving on as you need to move on in that way which is natural and of value .... memories now kept like jewels .... pretty, and of value, which can be taken out for a time and worn .... that enhance and make splendid, as their light reflects and makes special all that is there .... and you will be there with those jewels that are yours to keep.

Please take some time now .... time to spend with that person who is here with you now .... some private and special moments .... while I wait back here for you .... to let me know when you have completed all that you can there .... resolving any remaining problems and are ready to let go .... by just saying " I have finished here".

(Wait until the client responds)

That's good .... now you need to tell that person how much you love them .... and say that last good-bye for now .... feel the love that you will carry with you .... that feeling of peace and calm inner wisdom that is yours from your experience .... go ahead now, hug that person .... and say that last good-bye .... now.

And now that person returns .... is gone now .... leaving with you that wonderful feeling of peace within .... calmness of spirit .... a sense of renewed purpose as you now drift upwards, slowly reorienting to conscious awareness, bringing with you that new feeling of balance .... harmony .... and peace .... and when you will .... your eyes will open, and you can know that what has been done here will strengthen you more each day.

Float Away Stress

As you go deeper now .... each easy breath relaxing you .... calming you .... you can be aware of how comfortable and peaceful you are becoming .... as your body relaxes and your mind relaxes with it .... all tension .... all anxiety and fear just draining away now and calm filling you completely.

I would like you to imagine that you are in a sailing boat, all alone, floating on a lake .... all around are mountains, their steep sides covered with forests of pine trees .... their peaks snow-capped.

You have sailed to the very centre of the lake, enjoying the fresh crispness of the air and the scent of the pine forests carried on the breeze that drives the boat .... filling the sails at a gentle but exhilarating pace .... the splash and gurgle of the water as the boat cuts through the gentle swell .... the creaking of the rigging and the crack of the sails as they fill with each gentle gust of air.

You can be aware of how good you feel .... alone with your own thoughts .... alone with the sounds of nature all around .... a calm natural peace that knows no concerns or troubles .... nothing disturbs that peace .... nothing bothers you at all.

Now the wind drops to almost nothing .... the sails flap limply as they empty of the wind that drives the boat forward .... the surface of the water becomes calm .... still .... flat as a mill pond .... the surface ruffled only now and then by a gentle zephyr.

You feel the sun warming your skin .... comfortably warm .... soothing and relaxing you .... the quiet surrounds you now, broken only by the gurgle of water beneath the hull .... the faint sounds of birdsong .... the occasional splash as a fish rises to take an insect .... calm .... peaceful tranquillity surrounds you and envelops you.

You lie down on a soft cushion on the bottom of the boat, unconcerned at the lack of wind .... knowing that the engine is there and in perfect working order when and if required. You look up at the crystal clarity of the blue sky .... small clouds perfect and white hang above and around the tops of the mountains visible from where you are so relaxed and comfortable.

The still air carries the sounds of some fishermen .... casting their lines from the shore .... and there .... the distant tone of a church bell calms you .... relaxing you more with each note. High in the sky .... a jet trail marks the progress of an airliner .... etching its progress towards the far reaches of this wonderful world .... and you relax even deeper feeling within a calm, comfortable heaviness that is so pleasant .... so very nice.

The boat drifts .... rising and falling with the almost non-existent swell .... you are looking now at the very tip of the mast as it sways gently .... it appears to touch the clear blue sky above .... the air is so clean here .... you can taste it and you feel the calm tranquillity .... absorb that gentle peace .... and you drift too with thoughts that are pleasant and calming .... you breathe in peace and calm with every gentle breath .... breathing out anxiety and stress.

Here you have time to reflect on those things that have caused you stress .... you have time now to assess carefully and with a clarity never before available to you .... the importance and the relevance of so many different things. You realise that you have fallen into a habit of reacting in a manner which has proved stressful for you. You have reacted to stress in the same way that a bull responds to a red rag or to the matador's cape. You resolve now to ignore the red flags and to calmly reflect and decide on the most peaceful and effective way to live your life .... calmly .... confidently..... in control .... knowing that you are in control of you and of your life.

Things that are stressful are so because we allow them so to be .... and you are now that person who is aware that you do have the choice .... you choose to be calm and unaffected by the rush and hurry .... to make unhurried and calculated decisions that are the right ones for you and those who are important to you.

You can be aware now of the peace .... the calm .... the confidence that fills you .... expanding within you .... and you enjoy the stillness .... the warmth of the sun .... the subtle sounds of nature all around .... the sights and the scents that can allow you to be aware of the larger world .... the depth of water beneath you..... the natural world at peace with itself .... as all troubles and cares fade into unimportance .... insignificance.

You feel so much stronger now .... aware that the strength comes from deep within you .... it was there all the time .... hidden for a time beneath turmoil and stress, but now no longer shrouded within a veil of negativity and lack of confidence, it shines through .... and you recognize the strength that is yours and resolve now to use that which is yours to your highest benefit.

As the boat drifts you know that it can be so easy to allow the prevailing winds to take you wherever they will .... but in your vessel you have the power when winds blow, to tack and to steer, using the winds as you choose to guide which is the right way for you .... and you have in reserve, too, that engine .... that power which can mean to you that you have complete choice in the way you go .... but it can be pleasant to drift .... knowing that you can choose freedom .... calm .... confidence and you will, will you not?

If ever you feel burdened and stressed .... you can choose to get into your boat and drift whenever you need to, whenever you want to .... using the strength that is yours, and so growing stronger and stronger with every day.

Anger & Depression

And as you relax more and more, you can know that how we feel about something imagined or real, ... is really up to us.

It's like the man I once knew who bought a car .... brand new .... his pride and joy .... and he polished it and waxed it .... vacuumed the inside at least once a week, sometimes more .... He was so proud of that car .... until one day another driver reversed into it and put a huge dent in the side .... scraped the paint work, and he was so upset and hurt that he flew into a rage at first .... he refused even to drive the car for a week .... and when he finally did drive it .... he drove it like a lunatic .... thrashing the engine and crashing the gears .... and he refused to clean it or polish it .... and every time that he saw that huge dent .... a big deep depression in the side .... he became so very angry and sad .... and sometimes he even cried.

It changed his whole life .... nothing seemed to make him happy any more .... nothing seemed like fun.

He kept looking at that dent .... which reminded him how upset he was .... how angry .... every time he saw it he felt a twinge inside .... and he thought to himself .... "Why bother? .... Why me? .... Nothing ever goes right anyway!!"

The dent began to rust .... and after a while it became an ugly hole that he glanced at every day and felt that sad .... mad feeling again.

After a while .... he just didn't want to go anywhere .... didn't want to do anything, because each time he went out .... he saw that hole again .... and felt bad again .... just as though he wanted to go inside and hide.

It was as if he wanted to feel bad .... he felt as if he had a right to .... and he was right .... but he could have done something .... because he did have insurance, unlike the people who live in areas prone to floods .... who live next to rivers or by the sea .... where everything washes away when the river overflows its banks .... or the tide comes in further than normal .... they lose everything they have .... but move back when the waters recedes .... telling others that they are just glad to be alive.

I suppose it's hard to be mad at a river or the sea .... to take a flood personally. They just call it "an act of God" and go to church to pray that it will never, ever happen again .... but they know that it most probably will .... because rivers flood and the tide rises .... just as people make mistakes or do things wrong .... It's just their nature .... the way they are, and nobody thinks that a river or the sea should be different .... or gets angry when it does what it does .... and nobody worries that they caused the rain or the high winds that caused the flood.

They just move back in and get on with their lives .... and go swimming or boating .... glad that the sun is back .... the damage undone.

Now *(client's name)*, ... whether you like it or not .... it's entirely up to you .... but if you really want to feel better .... perhaps you can pay closer attention to what you think and what you do .... because you can choose to think about things that make you feel good .... that make you sad and feel bad .... or you can begin to do things that make you feel good. .... It's entirely up to you.

You can think sad thoughts .... you can remember bad feelings, or you can replace them with a comfortable participation in things that you enjoy.

You create the space in which you live. .... You have the ability to learn how to direct your thinking in whatever way you choose.

You can change what you do .... you can do things for you.   And so tonight .... tomorrow .... this week .... what I want you to do is this: .... every evening .... when you eat your evening meal .... your unconscious mind can automatically remind you .... perhaps with a particular sound .... a particular thought .... a particular image .... a stop sign of sorts .... an alarm .... that this is the time for you to decide what you will do that evening.

You can either decide to do something interesting, or something fun for a change .... or you can just decide to sit and think hard about every unpleasant thing .... about everything maddening event that has happened to you and about how upset you want to be about it.

It's completely up to you .... to enjoy yourself doing something different .... or to practise making yourself feel bad.

Self-Assertion

Direct approach for those who have lost sight of the priorities of life, and of their own abilities to make choices for themselves:

As you go deeper now, drifting to wherever your subconscious will take you, to a place where there is only peace .... calm .... and tranquillity .... and nothing concerns you other than the relaxing sound of my voice .... you can be aware that there really is no reason at all to make an effort to try to hear or to understand each and every word that I might say or not say .... Here .... as you rest quietly .... over There .... and it can be a comfort for you to know that your subconscious will hear and will understand everything that is important to you .... and it's so much easier to just allow those things to occur in their own way, while your conscious mind can drift to somewhere else entirely.

As you drift ever deeper with your own thoughts in your own way .... I would like you to pay close attention to each time I say the word .... NOW .... this will be for you a signal to go deeper still.

Many people come here to seek help with problems such as you are experiencing, and they will tell me I have no motivation .... no spark .... no zest, and my answer to them is always the same .... you have all the motivation you need, and that spark, that zest for life that once you found so readily available, is still with you, but it has become hidden .... lost within a mist of negative thoughts. But you can congratulate yourself right NOW on the fact that you found the motivation necessary to make the appointment .... and the spark of positivity to arrive here on time .... unlike that person who did not make the appointment .... did not have the motivation to make the effort .... that person is not here NOW .... sitting comfortably there .... that person was unable to distinguish the place from where they are NOW from the place where they would like to be.

You have all the motivation .... all the spark and the zest for life that you need, but there is one thing that you don't have .... yet .... and that's self-confidence .... the self confidence that it takes to set out on any journey or tackle any task, knowing that you have made all necessary arrangements and preparations .... knowing that you can .... you will .... complete that journey or that task .... easily .... quickly and without effort.

As you go deeper NOW .... please allow your subconscious to show you yourself at your place of work .... see yourself as you start your daily round of tasks .... NOW taking time to organize and prioritize those things that must be done. See yourself calm .... confident as you begin the first of those tasks, now taking the time .... seeing that task through to completion before beginning the next on your list of priorities.

If for some unforeseeable reason the task that you have begun cannot be completed, you remain positive as you complete that task as far as you are able and then set it aside, knowing that you have done all you can and that you can proceed no further until those elements required are available to you. It now becomes a new task, and you can, without hesitation or feelings of inadequacy or guilt, continue with the next of your priorities.

Should you be disturbed from the task that you are attending to, perhaps as a colleague requires your attention to what he or she considers important and wishes to be attended to immediately, you will be aware of a deep inner calmness that comes from deep within your subconscious .... helping you to feel calm and confident as you listen attentively, and in a calm, confident manner assess for yourself the importance of the situation .... and then, as those feelings of confidence and calmness grow stronger and stronger with every moment, ... see yourself NOW asserting yourself as calm and confident .... as you make your decision .... make your conclusion as to the importance and action required.

You are NOW comfortable and calm as that person who relies on you and has confident in the knowledge which you carry within .... confident in your own ability as you exercise your calm orderly approach to everyday tasks .... as you do this .... others appreciate you more, and their confidence in you grows as you exercise these special qualities of quiet calm and confidence.

You will experience more each day the satisfaction and the self- pride that attend your new and confident manner .... and those things that in the past caused you anxiety and feelings of inadequacy are NOW easy and of no concern. You will be pleasantly surprised at how easy they become, for you NOW accept that things do not need to be difficult and hard to warrant merit.

Each new task and each new challenge is for you NOW a pleasure, because you are aware of the simple and absolute truth .... the truth that you are at your best when you are relaxed, and that the most that anyone can expect of you is that you do your best.

You can NOW be aware also that even champion athletes who strive for perfection can make mistakes and sometimes get it wrong .... and even as they do their best .... that perfection, that great ideal is so seldom required or expected. A mistake is simply an opportunity to do it better next time.

You are NOW that person that you wish the world to see .... aware NOW of your own true value as a unique and special person, looking outward from yourself to those around you, aware that you have all you need to be certain that the decisions that you make for yourself are the right decisions for you and for those who are special to you.

You NOW take the decision to be responsible and caring for yourself, for you know that in this way you can be at your best and give of your best for those whom you love and care for, and who love and care for you .... and as you do this, your true personality will shine through .... others will warm to you and the bonds will grow stronger as your relationships grow and develop. You are calm, confident .... self-assured .... your personality, once dimmed within that mist of negativity, now shines brightly as those mists dissipate .... and that spark grows bright and clear for all to see .... bright and positive.

Experience NOW that good feeling, that positive and confident feeling that is yours as you choose to make the right choice for you .... as your subconscious mind does its best work for you without the need for you to know just how it knows what to do.

You now take quality time to be with those whom you love and who love you, time that means for you that only they are important whilst you are sharing yourself .... and to them you give this time freely.

From this time forward, your subconscious will remind you, as it can, of those things that are important .... that life is for living, and that work is part of that life which can also be enjoyed .... but always that you work to live and do not live to work. You now work to enjoy the justifiable rewards of your efforts, and gone forever is that feeling that tells you that you must feel guilty whenever you find pleasure in life, with your family and friends.

You NOW accept fully and without reservation that your subconscious mind will take care of you and all that is important .... and will remind you with a calming constancy of those things that have lasting and durable value .... that are significant .... and you NOW become a friend of your own inner friend and confidant that you are NOW intensely aware of

.... a wise and personal advisor deep within, with your best interests and well-being always the main consideration and motive. You NOW hear clearly and unmistakably the voice of that inner advisor .... that long lost friend and you renew that friendship, a close contact now always to be retained.

From this moment forward, you are your own person .... you NOW like, respect and love yourself more .... not in an egotistical way, but in a way that is beneficial to you as you listen to your own wise inner advisor and trust him/her to be with you at all times whenever needed.

NOW I want you to take in a deep breath, and as you expel all of the air from your lungs, go deeper NOW .... and as you turn inward to contact your own inner self, you can experience those new feelings of confidence and self esteem, that inner trust that allows you to know that you have all that you need to be the person that you wish to be as those feelings expand and grow to cocoon you NOW within a glow of warming and calming influence that allows you to always be at your best .... positive .... confident .... self- assured .... motivated and full of the spark and the zest for life that is there within.

Age Progression

A utility for allowing the new subconscious patterns to be experienced in future contexts. This can be incorporated into many sessions to provide you with a check on your work.

And now that you have had the opportunity to discover something about yourself, I wonder how many ways you'll find to use this new ability of yours creatively on your own behalf .... and it can be as if a long time has passed since this session .... a few days .... and a few months ago that we spent some time together where you learned that you could feel so good .... and you had a thought at that time that allowed you to look at yourself differently .... and as you look back over the time that has passed since then, how has that thought affected you? What things are different? What can you do now that you couldn't do then? ....

Pin-Point

Regression technique:

And now .... as you drift deeper with the sound of my voice .... into that place of safety that you can choose .... nothing bothers you or disturbs you at all .... and while we, for the purposes of this therapy, begin to explore those memories of yours .... of significance and of value .... I want you to know that I am Here with you as you rest quietly There .... nothing can harm you at all .... you can experience now a feeling of calm .... of peace .... of tranquillity.

And now I would like you to allow your subconscious to show you a railway station .... a very special railway station, where the trains that run on the track can go forward in time and also backwards to times past .... to memories of events that have occurred and have been hidden from you .... memories perhaps that are hurting you now and causing you anxiety and pain .... those memories that when exposed to the light of conscious awareness .... and your new experience and ability to form more appropriate and beneficial perceptions .... will lose their power to harm ever again.

Now experience yourself on that station .... choosing the carriage in which you will travel on that special train that will take you on that journey to past memories that are so important to you.

As you settle into your seat .... you relax deeper .... as the train begins to move off backwards into time .... as if then was now .... now is then .... as the train gathers speed .... you look out of the window .... events experienced pass by .... remembrances like telegraph poles along the track .... some instantly recalled .... some distant and vague .... so many .... so fast now .... the train gathering speed .... hurrying to where your subconscious mind knows is your important destination .... that special and important event in time .... and you can notice now that the train is slowing .... the clatter of the wheels changing note as the images that pass your window become slower and more distinct .... and now the brakes are applied .... as your subconscious mind chooses the exact moment .... the time that is now as the carriage comes to a halt and the door opens .... you step out .... and things and events are clear .... there .... now .... and you can talk to me and tell me what is happening .... who is there .... why is this important ....

The client's responses will now determine the direction and nature of the therapeutic interventions which are appropriate to use

Enuresis In Children

Have the child bring along a favourite toy such as a doll or Teddy bear that they would normally take to bed with them.

Hello *(child's name)* .... do you know why Mummy has brought you to see me today? Well, what we are going to do is play a little game that I know .... would you like that?

I see that you have brought *(Teddy or dolly)* along to see me .... would you tell me his/her name?

I bet you play with him/her a lot, don't you? .... and I bet too that you are very good at pretending, aren't you? .... Would you like to play a game of pretend with me now? Good. It's very, very easy to play .... all you have to do is just sit there as still as you can and then close your eyes for me .... can you do that? .... Mummy is going to play as well and she is going to close her eyes as well .... and I want you to pretend just as hard as you can .... that you just can't open your eyes at all .... and you can pretend so very hard that even if you want to open them .... you just can't .... and when I want you to open your eyes .... you won't be able to until I say special magic words .... When I say "Teddy says 'Open your eyes'", then you will be able to open your eyes .... but if I don't use those magic words then your eyes will shut tighter and tighter until I say "Teddy says 'Open your eyes'"...... and that's because you are pretending so well .... better than anyone else can .... that's very good.

Now as I talk to you about something very important, you can hear all of my words, but they all help you to pretend even harder than before that your eyes just will not open until I say the magic words .... and you can feel so nice and comfy sitting there in my comfortable magic chair .... nothing worries you at all .... and perhaps you can notice that you feel a little sleepy .... just a little bit .... so cosy there .... so warm .... cuddling Teddy now .... and, as I talk to you, you can think about something very important to you .... it's about that little problem that you have been having when you go to sleep in your cosy bed .... that you are so cosy and warm that you sometimes forget to remember that you need to wake up when you need to wee wee *(use the term most often used by the child)* .... you just forget to wake up and you have an accident that makes you feel so sad .... and then Mummy has to come along and change all of your bedclothes because they are all wet and uncomfortable for you .... and you really do want to remember not to forget to remember when it's so important .... don't you? .... I know that you think it would be so much better to remember not to forget .... and remember when you need to wake up and go to the toilet .... and you wouldn't even need to wake Mummy .... wouldn't it be good if you could do that every time?

Now I think that you could need just a little help from a very good friend of mine who helped me when I was a little boy, to learn how to remember to not forget to wake up in time .... and he has come here today to help you too .... he is going to show Teddy just how to help you remember every time that you need to go to wee wee .... and do you know .... he's so good at this .... you can be sure that you will never ever have that problem ever again.

My friend's name is Tommy Tinkle and he comes from a long way away .... where all of the fairies and the elves and the gnomes come from .... it's a place where all of the magic in the world comes from .... very, very special.

Tommy is five hundred and two years old .... and he even knows Santa Claus .... he helps him at Christmas to make sure that all of the children in the world get their presents on time .... he works very hard.

In a moment I'm going to call Tommy, and he has promised me that he will come here by magic to see you today .... all I have to do is say "Tommy Tinkle from over the moon, grant my wish and be here soon", and he will come right away .... but only you and I will be able to see him .... and only while our eyes are shut tight .... I am going to call him now.

"Tommy Tinkle from over the moon, grant my wish and be here soon."

My, that was quick .... he is here already, and as you are pretending so well, you can see him sitting in front of you on a little stool. He is funny looking, only as big as Teddy and just look at what he has on: .... a little red jacket with lots of silver buttons .... bright green trousers .... and yellow shoes with big buckles on the toes .... and what a funny pointed hat .... he even has a curly feather in it .... and he looks so very happy .... always laughing because he likes children very much. .... I wonder if you can count the buttons on his jacket .... how many are there? .... that's very good ....

Now (*child's name*), say hello to Tommy .... and I will tell you what he is going to do .... that he did for me when I was a little boy and found it so hard to remember to wake up in time to go to wee wee in the toilet .... a friend of my Mummy's asked Tommy Tinkle to come along and help me to remember to wake up in time .... you see, I had a teddy just like yours .... and Tommy showed my teddy just what to do and gave him some magic so that he would know just when I needed to wake up .... to go to the toilet .... to wee wee .... and I never ever had a nasty wet bed ever again .... I was so pleased and my Mummy was pleased too because she never had to get up to change those wet sheets ever again .... now he's going to do that for you .... and he is going to come over there and whisper in Teddy's ear the magic words that will help him to make sure that you always remember .... because teddies never ever forget magic words.

He will be very careful as he climbs onto the chair beside you .... so that he can whisper in Teddy's ear .... it won't take very long now .... so that Teddy will know exactly what to do for you .... Have you finished now Tommy? .... that's good .... he's nodding to me because I can't hear him like Teddy can .... perhaps you can hear him .... I know that when I was little I could hear him, but now that I'm grown up I can't .... because only children can talk to elves and hear what they say.

Now Teddy is going to show you what he has learned .... he knows exactly what to do .... and what to say to help you remember that you need to wee wee in the night .... but you must remember always to take him to bed with you .... and I know that Mummy will remember too .... Teddy is showing you now what he is going to do to wake you up .... what's he doing to you *(child's name)? (Wait for response, such as "He is pulling my hair" .... or "Tugging my nose" .... "Shouting in my ear")*. That's wonderful .... that is exactly what my Teddy did to me .... Now Tommy has to go because he is very, very busy .... so say "thank you" to him and "good-bye" now. "Good-bye Tommy, good-bye."

Now Teddy knows what to do .... and what to say .... he has all of the magic to help you never, ever forget .... now you can take him home .... and you will always remember to take him to bed with you every night, then he will be there to wake you when you need to wee wee, and you will never, ever have a nasty wet bed ever again .... so you will remember .... won't you?

You have been so very good at pretending and playing this little game with me, that Tommy has asked me to tell you that he is going to speak to Santa Claus and tell him just how good you have been .... and he is going to tell the tooth fairy to leave you something very special when she comes to see you.

Now I am going to say those magic words so that you can open your eyes and be very happy and proud at being so clever at pretending here with me today. "Teddy says 'Open your eyes'."

Flyaway

Script for fear of flying.

And now as you relax and go deeper .... I would like you to imagine that you are at an airport .... that you are here at the airport because you are going on the holiday of a lifetime to .... (*insert chosen destination*). You have packed all you need for the journey and for your holiday .... visas are all in order .... passports are safe and you have the tickets for your journey safe and secure.

I want you to notice that you are feeling calm and confident .... you are relaxed, and have only a small and understandable anticipation and concern .... appropriate feelings towards the coming adventure.

All around you are people arriving and departing .... to and from all the exotic and not so exotic parts of this world .... You hear strange languages .... see colourful and interesting national costumes as the people hurry to and fro.

The atmosphere is of calm and practised efficiency .... people moving through the terminal .... all possible problems have a solution .... everyone and everything is taken care of, and all arrive and depart efficiently and calmly .... so much order .... so many potential problems anticipated .... the solutions readily to hand.

You now move to the desk where you will check in your luggage .... and you are aware of the procedures to ensure that all baggage is checked and weighed ....x -rayed before being allowed to be stowed away in the aircraft that will deliver you to your destination.

And all the while .... the captain and his crew are checking the aircraft systems as they do before any flight .... they check every small thing in a specific and detailed manner .... in accordance with the check-lists that are standard to the aircraft .... check lists that have been developed through many thousands of hours of experience of the technology which is ever evolving through the years.

The captain will check that everything is as it should be, because he is aware that things can go wrong .... he has natural and professional caution and has learned that the systems that he depends upon are the best that can be relied on .... he checks because he is aware that thousands of aircraft fly millions of miles each day without mishap, as all of the captains check each and every flight, because they, too, want to be as sure as they possibly can that everything is okay .... he has confidence in the engineers who service the aircraft in accordance with strict schedules and limits .... confidence in the technology that he has to support him .... so much confidence because he spends so much of his life flying others from place to place across the globe .... but he reserves for himself that natural and appropriate respect for those things that can be checked and, when he has checked them, the confidence to know that he has done his work well .... left nothing to chance, and that he will arrive safely and without fuss, just one amongst many who fly the world almost without being noticed at all by those of us who travel only now and then .... every mile is logged and every second recorded as the journey continues .... a vast and international network .... working to international rules that all must comply with and adhere to .... and thereby safety is assured .... and the captain too must be checked .... he must pass inspection and he is subject to regular and stringent health checks every six months.... performance checks .... carefully monitored to ensure that he is fit to fly .... and I wonder if you are aware that when flying, both he and his co-pilot by regulation must be served different meals, to ensure that if the food is tainted, ... there will always be a qualified and capable pilot in charge of the aircraft.

Every system on the aircraft has a back-up system .... sometimes even three or more .... and you will be pleasantly surprised at how calm and confident you will be as you board the plane .... as you are shown to your seat .... aware of the quiet efficiency of the cabin crew as they ensure that you are comfortable .... just one more flight for them in their busy schedule .... and their air of calm and confidence will allow you to become more and more calm and more confident .... feeling safe and secure.

But you will experience .... and you will be aware of a natural and appropriate anticipation .... the anticipation that you feel whenever you undertake a new and exciting adventure .... enjoying the thrill .... enjoying the thrill of the anticipation of that new experience .... and you will be aware of a voice from deep within your subconscious .... a voice telling you that all is well and it really is all right to feel okay .... the voice of your own inner advisor .... that part of you that has perfect knowledge, and you can feel safe and secure in the knowledge that your inner advisor has all the knowledge that it needs to feel satisfied with the situation and will allow you to feel at ease .... safe .... excited .... and secure .... to see things in a different light, a warm and comfortable light that allows a feeling to change .... to rearrange those thoughts and images ....

allowing the mind to foresee that change in the future .... and to enjoy noticing as that future change occurs.

You will enjoy your flight and look forward with pleasure to a new experience .... always aware of the fact that you have perfect knowledge and your own wise inner advisor to remind you to exercise normal and natural appropriate caution in all things.

Fast Allergy Cure

Step 1: *Ask client to explain how he/she feels when having an allergy attack. Get him/her to describe all symptoms.* What happens to you? Where are you? What do you hear, see and feel?

Step 2: *Instruct the client to close his/her eyes. Then:* I want you now to think about when you are having an attack, to experience all of those uncomfortable sensations as you are having that attack. *(Reiterate the symptoms and discomforts obtained from step one).* Now pump up all of those feelings and symptoms. Make them as strong as you can. *Anchor, by touching the back of the client's hand.* .... Now let those feelings pass.

Step 3: *Ask the client to open his/her eyes and explore the feelings and sensations.*

Step 4: *Ask the client to think of something pleasant. Then ask him/her to describe the sensations and feelings when he/she is not suffering an allergy attack, when things are normal.*

Step 5: *Describe the operation of the immune system. Describe the presence of marker cells whose job it is to identify harmful objects such as germs and viruses that have entered our body, and killer cells whose job it is to latch on to and destroy foreign organisms. When someone develops an allergy, the immune system is mistakenly triggered into action by a benign substance which it then marks and attacks, causing an allergic reaction.*

Step 6: *Ask the client to again close his/her eyes. Then continue:* Now imagine that it is the sort of day when conditions are such that you will suffer an allergy attack. Now as you sit so comfortable and relaxed over there, I would like you to see right across the room in front of you. There is a solid, unbreakable glass screen, about four inches thick, and on the other side of that screen I want you to see *(client's name)* walking along with his/her immune system operating efficiently, the micropansies doing their work efficiently, marking the foreign bodies and the killer cells destroying them appropriately.

Touch back of hand (Anchor) .... Now notice how good you feel, and how well and appropriately your immune system is working for you. And now *(client's name)*, I want you to just float back into the room, here to where you are sitting. There, allow those good feelings and appropriate actions on the part of your immune system to integrate now, let those efficient and appropriate immune system reactions strengthen and integrate fully and completely.

Step 7:   *Now allow anchors to subside and carry out a test.:* If you were in that situation where you used to suffer from that allergic reaction; (*Describe situation, allow client time.*) tell me how you would be feeling now.

If you have been successful, the client will describe, feeling well and without the symptoms previously experienced.

Anxiety / Worry

Now that you are so very relaxed, your mind is receptive and open to new ideas .... ideas that will help you to stop worrying and enjoy life much much more.

Worrying is in fact looking into the future, predicting what might be, but focusing on only that which could go wrong.

When we care very much about someone .... or something .... it is no surprise when we worry; .... it's not pleasant, but it is natural and it is understandable. However, if there is no crisis, or when a crisis is over, we should stop worrying, relax, and enjoy life.

Because everyone needs to relax at times, even champion athletes who are under a great deal of pressure to perform, and sometimes need to be perfect to win, even they need some way to relax and to put things into perspective, to recognize that it is just a sport and not a war between nations. Because a war is one thing, and a game is something else entirely, especially in this nuclear age where a war could mean the end of everything. We really cannot afford to make the smallest of mistakes, and so some people are terrified that the fail-safe system will fail, and that will be the end of it, all because of some small error .... someone doing something wrong or saying something wrong at the wrong time, or to the wrong person, in the wrong way. Then everything goes up in flames.

Which is why they have special programmes for the people who are working with these systems, because what they have to do is so dangerous and terribly important that special training and counselling is required. This is probably the only place and situation in the world perhaps where mistakes cannot be allowed, and it is comforting to note that in almost every other place and situation, an error is just an opportunity to do it differently later on, because perfection is seldom needed and rarely required, and even champion athletes are never perfect all the time, and sometimes get it wrong. It is like the Navaho Indians who, when they weave their beautiful rugs and blankets, always leave a knot, an imperfection, so that the gods will not be angered and think that the weaver is trying to be a god.

But that is another story about what is really important and what is not, and how it feels to give yourself permission to enjoy the feeling of freedom to feel safe doing those things, knowing that the world will not end if you leave a knot somewhere, so that the gods will know that you are not challenging them, just doing the best that you can, and letting it go at that.

To overcome your tendency to worry, follow this simple two step formula:

1. First promise yourself that you will not worry about the small things.
2. Realise now that it's all small things.

We both know that you have an active mind and a reactive body, and if you think that scary thought for just one brief moment, then it has been scaring you. We also know that there are other things that you can think which are comfortable and calming, relaxing and reassuring thoughts or images that you can use instead, to help you to relax, to retain that relaxed, calm feeling.

You can let your unconscious mind learn all it needs to know to be able to distract you from those scary thoughts, to be able to provide you with those relaxing thoughts and images.

And I think that you will enjoy being happily unconcerned, unable to remember to worry in exactly the same way or at the same time. So from now on, when you enter that situation, you can enter it knowing that you are protected and can tell that part of you that tries to do its job by telling you that there are things to be afraid of here, that you really don't need it anymore. So it can either go away or find a different game to play, and remind you instead of all the good things that might happen here, or of all the fun things that might occur later, because those old thoughts and fears just aren't useful anymore.

So you can relax and forget it, go on about your business, surprised to discover perhaps that you have been thinking about something else entirely. And you will know at that point, deep down in every cell of your being, that you won't ever have to feel that way again, that it is over and done with, more rapidly than you expected. You can do it now and you can do it later, you can frighten yourself with that thought, or you can calmly relax yourself with a different thought. That's right, ... so practise and choose, it all belongs to you.

That Quiet Inner Voice

with clients who need to become aware of their own capabilities and gain con, *ence in their own inner awareness and capacities for self determination.*

As you continue .... drifting .... deeper with each breath that you take .... you can be aware of how little you need to be aware of .... the sounds in the room .... the ticking of the clock perhaps .... the rustle of papers .... sounds outside .... Each sound helps you to relax even more deeply .... each word that I utter is just a signal for you to become less and less aware of the importance of all that is unimportant here .... the exact meaning of words that are said or not said as I talk to you here .... nothing bothers or concerns you as your conscious mind drifts off to a place which is comfortable and safe .... and your unconscious mind takes on the responsibility for guiding and directing your awareness .... down .... into your innermost self .... aware now of that gentle connection .... communication with that part of you that is the essence of you .... that knows all .... remembers each and every event that has served to shape and mould your unique and special personality .... a part of you that you really do hear as a quiet and calm voice from within .... a voice of wisdom and of truth that is so often lost within the clamour and the clatter of the world .... the demands .... the constraints .... the noise that is those who would have you bend to their will .... now hear that voice still, quiet and calm .... but now clear as crystal .... piercing through the fog of indecision and lack of confidence .... unmoved and unaltered in its determination to give to you at all times .... good council .... wise answers and solutions to all problems .... to your highest benefit and of those who are special to you.

This is that creative and special part of you .... that wise inner advisor that is always there for you with your benefit and well-being always the prime consideration .... a constant, etheric part that is you and was you before there was awareness of this existence in this time .... an invaluable friend that must be listened to .... and you will, will you not?

You can recognize now that value, that unique capacity and capability that is yours .... has always been yours .... and I really don't want you to know too much how good you can feel with that intense awareness of confidence in your ability to make changes and decisions in your life for yourself .... no longer allowing others to manipulate you .... to take advantage of you .... you expect of yourself everything that is yours .... that you deserve .... that you are entitled to as a unique and special person .... aware of who you are .... aware of your own talents and special qualities .... always that person who is the forefront .... always there with a valuable input to every situation .... you listen and take note of what is important, and then you make a decision .... you make your own decision, and are comfortable in that.

I wonder if you can notice soon how others will come to rely on you to be the person that you are .... confident and self-assured .... an example to those who will admire you as you allow those qualities so long hidden .... to burst forth from within .... to astound and confound those who would manipulate and control .... you are your own person .... proud .... confident .... taking responsibility for your own life and well-being .... a true friend of your own wise inner advisor .... that is you personified.

Confidence-Building

Firstly *(client's name)*, ... I would like to extend my congratulations on your decision to seek help and to allow yourself the experience of coming here today. I appreciate that you made the effort to make an appointment and to arrive on time.

Already now .... you know that you can do that ... it is in fact easy to do .... and what about that feeling of achievement .... how it feels to realise that what was easy first time, will be even easier in the future .... for it is from positive experience that you learn how to use your confidence in a way that builds and grows stronger every day .... increased self-worth .... recognising even more than before that only good and positive thoughts are of value to you .... negative thoughts harm you .... you allow only good and positive thoughts.

It's so very easy to be that person who does not allow for mistakes to be made, and it can be a comfort to know that an error is simply an opportunity to do it differently next time.

Perfection is almost never needed, and even those champion athletes are never perfect all of the time .... and sometimes get it wrong. .... It's interesting to observe that when the Navaho Indians weave their beautiful rugs and blankets, they always leave a knot .... an imperfection .... so that the gods are never angered and think that they are trying to be gods themselves.

It can be comforting to know that you can give yourself permission to feel safe and enjoy those things that are important, knowing that the world will not come to an end if you leave a knot .... so that the gods know that you are not challenging them. Just doing the best that you can and leaving it at that.

As you go deeper now, just listening to the sound of my voice .... you can be aware of those comfortable heavy feelings of legs, of arms, of the entire body that seems to float in time and space .... those hypnotic sensations that allow you to know that you have travelled from one state of awareness into another state in a calm and confident way. And I wonder now if you can allow those feelings to continue .... those comfortable, relaxed sensations of mind and body .... as you drift and dream .... and my voice drifts with you.

You now look to the future in the way that tells you that things will go well .... that you will succeed .... that you are special .... attractive .... intelligent and capable .... In this way, you program yourself to succeed and you will succeed. You now look to the future and see only good things and good people happening to you as you move forward to grasp opportunities .... seeing those opportunities, clearly .... intensely aware that all of your worthwhile goals are attainable.

You have all the confidence you need to build upon, all the capabilities and capacities to be that person that you want to be, special and exciting. You and you alone have your best interests at heart, you now take control of your life. Now .... you are taking control .... you trust your own judgement in all things and you know that you alone have your best interests, and the best interests of those who are close to you, within your control .... and it is with profound satisfaction now that you undertake and commit yourself to your own best interests, utilising to your highest potential, YOUR capability, YOUR special qualities, accepting YOUR feelings of self congratulation as you achieve your worthwhile goals.

You find it easy to concentrate on what is important to you .... your subconscious mind helps you in those ways, reminding you of your successes, of your positive abilities, of all your special qualities. Others appreciate you more as you demonstrate your confidence. Your positive approach allows those around you to have confidence in you, as your confidence grows and manifests itself in your day-to-day success. Now your creativity discovers new ways of releasing itself, to become effective and part of your own special personality. You impress and amaze all with your clarity of thought and expression of new ideas and input to every situation. Once the bystander .... now at the forefront, establishing yourself as that interesting positive person that you are. You can now .... be aware that you are the equal of all, relaxed and comfortable in every situation. You are realising, now with greater clarity each and every day, that you can unlearn that feeling of fear and lack of confidence. You now take a deep breath, relax yourself from head to toe, and take the image into your mind of you .... happy and secure .... confident and self-assured, as you tell yourself .... I CAN .... I WILL. This comfortable, pleasant image soothes your mind, and all fear and self-doubt leave you completely.

You unlearn fear by being positive and realising that the only thing that can hurt you, is the fear itself. No longer do you accept fear or negativity, you banish in their entirety all unwanted, inappropriate thoughts and symptoms, allowing only good thoughts and positive feelings to grow and become part of your special personality. You do this easily because you are in control. It will become easier and easier for you to do this as you take control, and you will take control, will you not? *(Await response.)*

As you go deeper now, in control, just listening to the sound of my voice, your subconscious mind shows you yourself at that time .... that place .... when you really felt confident, ... a time when you really felt good ..... when you were the centre of attention, loved and admired. Being congratulated by those around you as you received an award for achievement .... or realised a long-standing ambition. It doesn't matter where it was or when it was, just as long as you felt really good about yourself and about your achievement. Think of your finest hour, and get that image into your mind as you were at that time, at that place. You see yourself right now as the centre of attention, with all others cheering you .... congratulating you .... Now hold that feeling .... Allow that feeling to be something that you can expand. Now see that special feeling as a pulsating white light, warm and comfortable .... powerful .... allow that white light to expand and grow so that it encompasses you, so that you are completely contained within a brilliant cocoon of pulsating white light. Feel that warm and comfortable feeling .... confident and admiring thoughts about you and your special qualities and capacities. Feel it growing .... expanding, filling your very being with its power and positive influence. And now allow that white light to be absorbed into your body, as you absorb completely and permanently, to your highest benefit, all those good and capable qualities which ensure that from this moment forward, you are the confident and self-assured person that you want to be, that you are right now.

Each and everything thing you do, you do better than you have ever done before. You approach each new task with complete ease of mind knowing that you are relaxed and in a perfect frame of mind, ... calm .... relaxed and confident. Every day your confidence grows; .... that means that tomorrow your confidence grows and the day after it grows stronger than before. As you practise being more and more confident, so your confidence grows and becomes stronger as more and more .... your feelings of self-worth become strong and powerful. Each day, with each new situation .... whenever you need to, you take control, calm your mind, disregard troubles and you are calm .... relaxed .... poised .... competent .... and confident .... You are your own person .... is that not so?

(Wait for response and then go to trance termination)

Confidence Booster

As you become more and more relaxed and less tense each day .... so .... you will remain more relaxed .... and less tense when you are in the presence of other people .... no matter whether they be many or few .... no matter whether they be friends or strangers.

You will be able to meet them on equal terms .... and you will feel much more at ease in their company .... without the slightest feeling of insecurity or inferiority .... without becoming self-conscious or embarrassed in any way.

You will become so deeply interested .... so deeply absorbed in what you are saying .... that you will concentrate entirely upon this to the complete exclusion of all else.

Because of this you will remain perfectly relaxed .... perfectly calm and self-confident .... and you will become less conscious of yourself and your own feelings.

You will consequently be able to talk quite freely and naturally .... without being worried in the slightest by the presence of any other persons. If you should begin to think about yourself .... you will immediately shift your attention back to your conversation .... and you will no longer experience the slightest nervousness .... discomfort or uneasiness.

The moment that you get up to speak .... all of your nervousness will disappear completely .... and you will feel completely relaxed .... completely at ease .... and completely confident. You will become so deeply interested in what you have to say .... that the presence of an audience will no longer bother you in the slightest .... and you will no longer feel confused .... uncertain .... or conspicuous in any way.

Your mind will become so fully occupied with what you say .... that it will make you feel confident about what you are saying. Nervousness, feeling self-conscious or embarrassed will be but a memory of past behaviour .... because you will remain throughout .... perfectly calm .... perfectly confident and totally self-assured.

Self-Esteem Booster

Imagine that you are wearing a sign that tells the world "I am a unique and very special person". You always wear that sign .... that badge and you wear it with pride. Every day you become more and more aware of your assets and the qualities and beauty within you.

You now place your complete trust in you .... in your own inner mind .... the values and opinions that you accept are your own .... you make up your own mind .... you trust your own judgment .... opinions and values .... relevant .... informed and special.

Decisions that you have been putting off will be easier now because you trust you and your ability to make those decisions which are the right ones for you and those you love .... those who are special to you and rely on you and your special wisdom .... strength .... all those qualities and capacities are within you.

You admire yourself .... like yourself, and trust yourself so much more .... others too find it easy to like you .... to respect you .... to admire you .... to love you .... but you no longer worry or concern yourself about what others think of you .... it matters only that you like and respect yourself.

You are aware that you cannot please everybody and that the only way to be successful in what you do is to trust your own judgment and to please yourself .... what is right for you will be right for those who are close to you. As you do what is right for you .... always trusting your own judgment .... having that belief in yourself .... you now have the confidence to do what you want to do .... Those who would manipulate you and take advantage of your easy-going nature ..... are now confounded .... aware that with due consideration .... you do what is right for you and those who are important to you.

You trust your own judgment and meet your own special and legitimate needs and the needs of those who are close to you and who are special. You meet those needs .... you are independent and self-sufficient.

Changes are happening within you .... changes for the better .... some you will be aware of now .... others you will be unaware of until some time in the future.

As you trust yourself more and more .... your subconscious mind will cause these ideas to be made available to you .... ideas for your benefit.

These ideas will be absorbed for your betterment so that you can easily overcome any problem. Know and believe .... whatever the mind can conceive .... the mind can achieve. Whatever you believe you can achieve .... you will achieve. Every day you are feeling more and more comfortable within yourself and you are becoming your own best friend. Every day you love and respect yourself more, not in an egotistical way .... but in a way that is positive .... natural and constructive .... and can be only beneficial to you.

Take a moment now to enjoy the feeling of liking yourself and being happy and content with the unique and special person that you are.

Know and believe that each and every small part of your mind .... your body and your spirit is an important .... wonderful and beautiful part of nature. Spirit means your higher self .... that part of you which is inspired .... strong .... kind .... loving and happy .... all of those good and special qualities that are to be admired. Those special qualities are an integral part of your unique personality and are there for you whenever you need them. If there are things that you have done in the past that you regret .... now is a good time to forgive yourself. Forgive yourself now and release yourself now from the shackles of those negative elements which prevent you from moving forward. Now you can be that person that you want to be.

If there are any things which others have done to you in the past .... now is the time to forgive those others. Forgive others now and release yourself right now from the past .... you now live for the moment .... this moment. Now you are that person that you want to be .... a true friend of your own personal and wise inner advisor who is you personified.

The Filing Cabinet

For use in analysis to assist the client to access relevant memories, re-evaluate and dispose of uncomfortable repressions.

Now as you relax more and more .... each word that I utter is just a signal for you to go deeper now. We are going to be working directly with your subconscious mind.

You will recall that I have told you that every memory .... dream .... event in your life is stored in your unconscious mind .... good .... bad .... insignificant .... it's all there stored .... rather like a filing cabinet .... and now your subconscious will assist you here to go through that filing cabinet, seeking memories of importance to you .... of significance that relate to your problems .... memories .... feelings and emotions that will be beneficial for you to recall here in the course of your therapy.

Just relax .... deeper now .... and allow yourself to drift along one passage of your mind until you can see a faint outline .... of a grey door. As I count to three, with each count see it becoming clearer. 1 .... becoming clear now .... 2 .... clearer still .... 3 .... you can see it really clearly now .... as you draw nearer and nearer to that door. Closer and closer now .... reach out now and open the door .... now enter into the room beyond that door .... and close the door behind you.

You can see now that you are in a cream painted room .... well-lit and airy .... even though you cannot see the source of the light, you will see everything. In the centre of the room is a plain, wooden table .... to the side of the table is a tall filing cabinet with four grey drawers .... and one black drawer at the bottom. There is nothing else at all in the room. As you walk over to the cabinet .... notice the label attached to the black drawer .... the red print says clearly .... not to be opened .... not to be read.

The grey drawers contains all of those day-to-day memories of your life .... mostly happy .... some sad .... everything that you have seen .... done .... heard .... or experienced; .... memories that are available to you at all times to help you with each new experience.

The black drawer however .... contains memories that your subconscious has decided to keep from you .... to hide from you .... and the answer to the problems that you have are there in that drawer .... that memory or memories that form for you the basis of so much hurt and pain .... so much misery. Within this drawer are those memories that, once shown to the light of conscious awareness, cannot be re-filed in a hurtful way .... or cause you problems ever again. Hidden away .... yes .... they caused you problems and pain .... but once brought out into that light of awareness they lose that power to cause you problems ever again, just as if they were never there.

You have come here to understand .... and to resolve your problems. By using this opportunity to examine those hidden files .... you can resolve them .... easily .... quickly .... and permanently. You cannot see your subconscious mind .... since it is formless .... but as you wait now by the table .... the black drawer will begin to slide open .... silently .... on well-oiled runners. As it slides open .... you can see the label on the drawer being removed as if by invisible hands .... torn in half .... and then dropped onto the floor.

You are now free to examine everything in the drawer. Look inside and you will observe a number of ordinary brown files. From here .... I can't see how many files there are in the drawer, but you .... there .... can see and you can count them now. Tell me *(client's name)*, how many files are there?

Inside each of these files is a piece of paper, or perhaps several sheets. Each sheet will have on it a word or words written or printed upon it, ... perhaps in black ink .... perhaps in coloured ink. You may find that some of the sheets have no writing at all, but a picture .... a drawing or a photograph which you will recognize and find easy to understand.

Now your subconscious is taking out the first file .... laying it open on the table .... handing to you the first page .... it is in your hands now. Look at it .... and tell me what you see.

There may be only one word on the page or it may be covered with writing or with pictures .... look at the page .... let what happens happen: .... you are looking at memories and they cannot harm you.

As you reach the end of the page, turn it over and examine the back .... there may be further detail.

What is on that page? It is no longer a secret .... dark and hidden .... no longer the unknown .... its power to harm you has gone .... it no longer has that power. Now that piece of paper is of no further use.

Lay it quietly on the table for your subconscious to dispose of safely .... in any way it sees fit. Then go and take out the next file.

(Continue until the client tells you that the drawer is empty).

Now that you have had this opportunity .... and you have seen all that was hidden away from you for such a long time .... you have been able to see and to understand what has been causing your pain. Now that you know what was there, it can no longer hurt you in that way and cause you problems ever again.

Now watch, as the drawer begins to change colour .... that deepest black now fading to become grey .... the same as the others .... now ready to store new and pleasant memories for the future.

Snapshots

This is a strategy to move client into accessing memories that are important during analysis.

Now in this relaxed and comfortable situation, your subconscious for your benefit will accept my suggestions which are for your benefit and welfare in the context of this therapy .... here as you listen to the sound of my voice and the words that I say or do not say here..... and each word relaxes you as you go deeper into relaxation with each word that I utter.

I would like you now to allow your subconscious to show you a room .... a well-lit room that is very warm and comfortable .... a room where you feel totally safe and secure .... in the centre of the room is a large table that is there for you .... and there is a comfortable chair there just for you .... now walk across to that chair and sit down and become ten times more deeply relaxed.

As you go deeper now, you can see that on the table, there is a large wooden document box, a very old box, and you will see that on the table, beside the box, there is a key to that box .... Now you can pick up that key and find that it fits the lock on that box perfectly, and it turns easily as you unlock that box.

Now look inside the box and find it full of mementos of your life .... there are albums filled with photographs of all manner of things .... objects, things that you will recognise, ... most of them unimportant .... but some of great importance to you, of significance and of value here. These are snapshots of your life, hidden for so long in the deepest parts of your subconscious memory; yes, they may have cause you pain and problems in the past, but now, exposed to the light of day and to your conscious mind, they lose their power to cause you pain.

It is for you now to take out those albums from that box. I cannot see how many there are, but I know that you are able to see clearly now, and find that special album of significant importance and value to you now, just one in particular that stands out now in some way that your subconscious will understand indicates that here within are the answers to your problem(s).

Find that album now and place it on the table in front of you. Now you can begin to examine the contents of that album, so open it up at the first page and then examine it carefully and tell me what you see that is of importance to you, of significance and of value. You can speak to me clearly but you cannot wake .... Now go ahead, aware that I am here to help you and that you are perfectly safe and secure. All within that album are but memories, they do not have any power to harm you in any way. Now tell me *(client's name)* .... what do you see here? .... what do you feel? .... what are you experiencing?

Continue to deal with each page and it contents in turn, and then, in a significant manner, have the client dispose of the material - tear it up, or throw it into the fire, or whatever seems appropriate. Ensure that any photographic negatives are also destroyed at the same time, and assure the client that he/she can be satisfied that no other copies exist.

The Three Doors

Strategy for eliciting repressed memories.

And now as you relax and go deeper .... please allow your subconscious to show you yourself Here standing There in a corridor .... You feel totally safe and secure .... the corridor is well-lit, although you cannot determine the source of the light. The floor is carpeted with a thick pile carpet, and you can be aware that the colour of this carpet is a colour that your subconscious knows to be relaxing. Tell me *(client's name)*, what colour is the carpet there?

You see that this corridor has three doors and that each of these three doors has a number on it .... 1 .... 2 .... or 3.

Behind each of these doors are kept all of your life memories .... not one single experience has been missed .... all are stored there .... here .... safely stored. Doors 1 & 2 are painted grey .... behind these doors are all of the ordinary memories of your life .... some happy, some sad .... all of the everyday ups and downs of life .... thoughts, images .... all of the emotions attached to each of those memories are there .... there for you to recall as experience .... wisdom ....likes and dislikes .... ways of doing things and ways of coping with each new experience that life offers you. Door 3 is different .... this door is painted the deepest black .... a door that has been for such a long, long time kept securely locked .... the key hidden from you by your own subconscious.

Hidden from your awareness are memories that are uncomfortable .... tragic .... black, guilty secrets .... memories of hurt and sadness .... of anger and frustration .... evil memories that, whilst hidden and secret, form the basis for so much hurt and misery for you. Behind that door lie the answers to problems that now affect the quality of your life .... memories whose power lies in the fact of their secrecy .... memories that will lose their power when that door is opened and they are exposed to the light of conscious awareness .... lose their power to hurt you and cause you problems ever again .... You will be free.

Your subconscious mind will now show you the key .... see it now floating in front of you .... and as you watch, that key moves to the lock and now in the lock .... it turns easily and silently, and that door slowly opens wide.

You are here .... in that corridor there to resolve your problems .... to understand .... and now you can enter into that room and resolve them easily and permanently. As you enter the room, you notice that the door remains open wide .... within this room is your unconscious .... you cannot see it because it is formless, but as you wait there for just a moment, it will reveal itself to you in some safe way that you will understand .... and it will reveal to you in some manner .... it may be visual .... a face perhaps or a familiar place .... or perhaps a sound .... a voice or even music .... it may allow you to experience its presence by way of a feeling .... but you will understand as it begins now to reveal to you the very source of your problems.

It may show you pictures .... or words .... a drawing perhaps .... maybe in colour, or in black and white .... a photograph perhaps .... whatever it is, you will know it and understand it. Whatever your subconscious mind shows you here .... is okay and safe for you to look at .... You are looking at memories .... so now look around the room and whatever happens .... just let it happen .... Whatever you are shown is right for you now to know about .... perhaps a secret exposed .... and because it is exposed .... its power to hurt you will be gone .... over, once and for all time.

Tell me what you see .... what you are experiencing as you enter into that room now.

I explain to the client that once they have dealt with all of the memories important to them in the room, the power of those memories to harm them will be negated. Once they are satisfied that they have done all that is necessary, I tell them to go out into the corridor and then to close the door. If they have done all that is required, then the door will close easily, but if there are still matters that need to be dealt with, then the door will not close. Tell them to go ahead, "Can you close the door?" If the answer is "No", then they have not finished, and they must go back to confront whatever is preventing them from moving on.

As your subconscious mind has revealed these secrets to you for your understanding .... I wonder now if you have noticed that the door is now beginning to change colour.... changing now to grey just like the other two .... the room is empty now and ready to store new memories .... positive and pleasant memories for the future.

Smoking Therapy

As a practising hypnotherapist, you can expect that a good proportion of those who come to you for help will be smokers seeking to quit their habit. Hypnotherapy has the reputation of being the best therapeutic help for smoking cessation available, with an excellent success rate.

When asked what the rate of success is, I always tell my clients that I am not able to be exactly accurate, as those who come to see me and who stop smoking will invariably forget to tell me in six months whether they are continuing not to smoke. The only really reliable indication I have is when a client is referred to me by another, and I have an encouraging number of those.

I have heard some therapists claim a 60% or 70% success rate, and some even higher, but how they are able to come up with these figures without indulging in a lengthy survey over several years, I am not really sure. I am sure that if I have two clients and both are successful, then I can quote, quite tongue-in-cheek, a success rate of 100%!

I find that it pays to be honest and sometimes quite blunt with people who call. It takes some nerve to tell someone who is going to pay you for the service you provide that, unless they really want to stop smoking, they may as well not bother wasting your time and their money. "If you really do want to stop smoking, then fine, I will make an appointment for you right now to come along, but I have to say this to you: if you are not sure whether you want to stop or not, but perhaps just thinking that you will come along and see if I can stop you, then please don't bother me and waste your money." *Make plain to your prospective clients that you need their full co-operation if you are to be able to help them to help themselves in that way.*

"How many sessions will I need?" *This can be the subject of some debate within the profession. There are differing views, but myself I work on a simple premise: provided that the client's smoking habit is not evidently part of the symptomology of some deeper and more complex problem, and can be safely defined primarily as habitual, then the problem can be resolved in just one session. If it doesn't work the first time, then it is not going to work. There are other factors at work here, and they need to be resolved before this coping mechanism can be dispensed with.*

During the initial interview and fact-finding exercise, you, the therapist, will be able to determine from the demeanour of your client whether or not you will have to deal with other factors before you can help your client to give up the symptom that is his/her smoking. This comes with experience, and that I cannot give you here.

My 'Stop Smoking' session begins with a discussion about the client's life-style, his/her family and relationships. I want to know about the stresses in his/her life; what is important; what frightens him/her; his/her aspirations and motivations: in essence, what are the controlling influences in their life.

I want to know how they started and when; what they remember about the first cigarette smoked; why they chose to continue when the first cigarette was so awful. The answers to these questions are usually pretty much the same. "Mum and Dad smoked, and it seemed to me that I could count myself grown up when I too began to smoke." "My friends all smoked, and it seemed to be the thing to do to be one of the crowd." *(Peer pressure).* "I started in order to annoy my parents and show them they couldn't tell me what to do". *Whatever the answers, they will invariably point to the association with being grown up, one of the crowd, more sophisticated and mature, establishing independence.*

What do you get from cigarettes? *Once again the answers are so predictable.* "It helps me to relax." "It helps me to concentrate." "It calms me down." "It's something to do with my hands." "It gives me an excuse to have a break."

I have yet to hear a declaration, "It make me smell nice and attracts people to me.", *or* "I will live longer and stay healthy longer." *or* "I really do need to get rid of this money that I would otherwise spend on luxuries and things that really matter."

I ask when they smoke, beginning with when they wake in the morning. Before breakfast, after breakfast, in the car, on the telephone, after a meal, with a cup of tea, and so on.

I ask questions such as, "Do you know of any person who has died from a smoking related disease, or do you know of someone who is at this time ill through smoking?" "What do your family and friends think of you smoking?" "Have you had any warning signs that your own health is suffering?" "Has your doctor mentioned your smoking?"

Much of the time, the answers to all these questions and more will emerge as the client begins to talk frankly, perhaps for the first time in his/her life, about the habit and what he/she knows to be the dangers and the social consequences.

In therapy, we use the fears and the aspirations of our clients to their profound good, as we project that danger and fear which is consciously recognized into the subconscious mind where the seat of the habit dwells.

In the foreword of this book, I have mentioned that the scripts contained within should be considered as adaptable. They are not a magic formula which, if incanted in the special circumstance of hypnotic trance, will instantly turn lead into gold. You will learn to utilize the special fears and motivations of your individual clients and build into the framework which is the script effective interventions appropriate to the circumstances present.

For a young woman of childbearing age, the importance of providing a good, rich supply of oxygenated blood clear and free of contaminants has to be a factor that can be used with effect. "Do you really wish to feed your baby on nicotine, arsenic, benzo-pyrene, carbon monoxide, etc."? *I am sure that by now you have caught my drift.*

As therapists, we see ourselves as members of a caring profession, but that does not mean that we must not use those aspects of smoking which are frightening. Indeed, it is sometimes necessary to show the full horror of what could be and to demonstrate what is eminently possible if the responsibility is not taken by the client for his/her own life and health.

The granny with her grandchildren can be reduced to floods of tears when she is asked in hypnosis to see herself not being allowed to hold her new-born grandchild. Similarly, the father given a suggestion that he is in a room with all his family around him and is instructed to tell them all that he has but a short time left to live, having contracted a smoking-related disease (the disease you have established to be the one he most fears), and to tell them all why. Whose fault it is that he will not be there for them?

We accentuate the guilt and the remorse, not because we are sadistic and take pleasure from the reaction that we invoke, but because we know that emotion is a very powerful driving force. After all, what is it that constitutes memory?

After the guilt and the remorse comes, the congratulations and the confidence-boosting, the sense of achievement and the knowledge that, from this moment forward, they will no longer be dependent on anything other than that which they possessed all along .... confidence and self-esteem generated from within.

When all around is chaos and unpredictable, we humans seek constancy and predictability, and it can be seen that, whatever else is happening and changing outside our control and influence, "a cigarette stays the same". A cigarette is constant, it is predictable, it does provide, at some level, a sense of constancy, and in this way can become a very potent influence. Therein lies the power of the habit.

I cannot emphasize enough the importance of tailoring your presentation of the script of the stop-smoking sessions to each client. Do carefully consider and use his/her fears and aspirations. This means of course, that you listen to what he or she is telling you as well as to what is being said.

I am including here a specimen questionnaire which will provide a basis for the initial interview. Once again, please accept it as a guide only. There are so many questions that could be asked, and so many answers that could be given. Every answer given has meaning that is particular to the person who is answering. To listen and hear really is the key.

Smokers' Questionnaire

Name: .... Age: .... Male/Female: ...... Date: ....
Address:..
....Tel:...............................
Occupation:..
Occupational Stressors: ....
....
Partner: .... Children: ....
Conditions within Relationship: ....
....
How many cigarettes etc. smoked per day?: ....
For how long?: ....

Why did you start?:　　　....... Peer pressure

　　　　　　　　　　....... Rebelling against authority

　　　　　　　　　　....... Mother and Father smoked

　　　　　　　　　　....... To appear more adult

　　　　　　　　　　....... To appear more sophisticated

　　　　　　　　　　....... Other

What do you get from smoking?

　　　　　　　　　　....... It relaxes me

　　　　　　　　　　....... It helps me to concentrate

　　　　　　　　　　....... It's an excuse for a break

　　　　　　　　　　....... It gives me a confidence boost

　　　　　　　　　　....... It's a prop

　　　　　　　　　　....... Other

When do you smoke?:　....... On waking

　　　　　　　　　　....... At breakfast

　　　　　　　　　　....... With tea

　　　　　　　　　　....... After meals

　　　　　　　　　　....... On the telephone

　　　　　　　　　　....... Whilst driving

　　　　　　　　　　....... At work

　　　　　　　　　　....... In bed

　　　　　　　　　　....... Other

What frightens you about smoking?:...
....
....

Do you know someone:
(a) who died from smoking related disease?...............................
(b) who is ill now? ....
Who is important to you?: ....
WHY?: ....
....
What else is important to you?: ....
....
Has your doctor mentioned your smoking to you?: ....
Have you had any warning signals or symptoms?: ....
Do you have any health problems?: ....
....
How long do you want to live?: .... Why?:...............
Whose responsibility is your health?: ....
What will you be able to do as a non-smoker that you could not do
before?: ....
....
What will you do with the money you save?: ....
....
Do you really want to quit?: .... What's stopping you?: ....
....
Observations: ....
....
....
....
....
....
....
....

Foetal Smokers

For use with expectant mothers, incorporate into Diamond Smoking Script.

Now as you go deep inside, you can be aware that, just as you have eyes that see the world about you, now closed and so relaxed .... you also have an eye which we can call your mind's eye .... and this eye is there for your subconscious to see all of those things which are so important to you now.

Your mind's eye is very powerful, and you can allow it now to show you deep within yourself a very special part where something miraculous .... something wonderful .... is occurring .... as you travel now where your perfect subconscious mind takes you .... as you go so very deep within .... you can be aware of a gentle yet powerful connection between your own creative and maternal self with another who is yet to be born .... growing within you.

I am now going to count from one to three, and with each count, your mind's eye will show you more clearly .... within your womb .... where your own child even now is growing .... nurtured and loved .... one .... becoming clear .... two .... clearer still .... three .... you can see quite clearly now that growing child within you and you can understand now the special communication that can be experienced now .... here is your child .... nurtured within you .... reliant on you for a rich supply of oxygenated blood full of nutrients, so that it may develop within you and grow healthy and strong, and I know that you can feel that special love now .... that desire to ensure that your baby has nothing less than the best that you can provide .... You eat all of the most nutritious foods .... full of vitamins .... healthy foods .... and you take so much care with what you drink .... aware of caffeine .... of alcohol .... of chemical additives .... their potential to harm your baby .... You determine now to commit yourself to being the best that you can be .... to ensure that your child is supplied with nutrient-rich oxygenated blood, free from contamination .... free from tar .... free from nicotine .... free from ammonia .... from benzo-pyrene .... free from carbon monoxide and from cyanide and from arsenic and from all the harmful and destructive chemicals contained in cigarettes .... And you can tell that child within you now of your love and your commitment to ensure that all is as it should be .... tell that child now .... and hear the voice of your child from deep within that creates a bond that will grow and become so powerful .... and should you wish, you can ask your child whether it will be born a girl or a boy .... and you can ask and be told so much .... so go ahead now while I just stay quiet for a few moments while you speak within privately .... and you can tell me when you are content that all is well .... just say "I am content".

(Wait for response and continue with stop smoking therapy.)

Diamond Smoking Script

Now as you relax, drifting deeper with every word that I speak, the first thing I would like you to know is just how much I appreciate and admire you for the decision you have made to give up once and for all this foul habit.

So many people come here for help with this problem; they say "I have no discipline .... I have no motivation." My answer to all of them is this: .... that person who has no motivation and no self- discipline did not come here today; .... that person is not sitting there, comfortable and relaxed in that chair; that person did not make an appointment, ... did not turn up on time, ... simply stayed where they were, not knowing the difference between where they are now .... and where they want to be. You have all the discipline that you need .... you have all the motivation that you need .... but, what you do not have .... yet .... is self-confidence. The self-confidence that it takes to set out on any journey .... or undertake any task, knowing that you have made all the preparations .... that you are completely prepared in all respects .... believing that you can .... that you will complete your journey or task easily .... quickly and without effort .... the same self-confidence it takes to recognize the signs of success .... just as you recognize now those comfortable hypnotic sensations .... perhaps a heaviness of legs .... or lightness of arms .... those physical signs that allow to you to know that you have moved from one state to another state in a calm and confident way. And in this calm and confident state .... you can offer yourself generous portions of self-confidence .... large helpings of self-esteem .... breathing out self-doubt as you relax even deeper and continue to enjoy the journey towards your goal.

Your conscious mind is fully aware of all of the dangers to health and to life that are the legacy of the tobacco trade; after all, there are enough warnings on television and in the press for all to see, ... there are even warnings from your caring government on the packets that you buy, ... and what about the obscene waste of hard-earned money that smoking signifies? Perhaps here .... now .... it is worthwhile to review the damage that is inflicted by you on your body each time you light up a cigarette.

Fact: .... in this country alone, over 500 people die an early death each day through smoking. Doctors attribute in excess of 450,000 heart attacks each year to smoking .... and although cancer would appear to be the most obvious health hazard .... and it is true that a smoker is 50% more likely to contract cancer .... It can be so easy to say, "It won't happen to me. Cancer happens to other people." Perhaps, then, it is right that we now consider some of the other ways that smoking can damage your health and even life itself.

The heart of a smoker works so much harder, beating up to 10,000 extra beats every day, as it struggles to combat the effects of nicotine .... restricting .... clogging .... closing up the arteries .... increasing blood-pressure as it strives to deliver oxygenated blood so necessary for the function of the vital organs of your body .... the muscles .... the brain.

You have told me that a cigarette helps you to relax .... Now I invite you to review and to question that statement in the light of knowledge that, in addition to the fact that your heart is working so much harder, each time you take cigarette smoke into your lungs, you introduce into your body in excess of 4,000 different chemical compounds, many of them deadly poisons .... none of them in any way beneficial. Your body reacts to these lethal poisons in the same way as when subjected to sheer terror .... the automatic response that we know as the "fight or flight response" is activated .... adrenaline production is elevated .... respiration increases .... blood pressure increases as the body prepares to fight, or to run away from danger. Nicotine .... Tar .... Ammonia .... Benzo-pyrene .... Carbon monoxide .... Arsenic .... Cyanide .. to name just a few, and what about the chemical fertilizers and the insecticides that are sprayed on the growing tobacco crops.... remaining to be included in cigarettes .... now absorbed into the tissues of your body?

Does this sound like relaxation? You know the truth, and this truth now becomes deeply embedded in the subconscious of your mind, not to be denied.

As your heart works harder, your lungs strive to perform their essential function. The inside of the lungs and airways are covered in tiny hair-like projections called scillia, and these become coated with thick sticky tar .... they become brittle and lie flat against the walls of the airways, now unable to perform their function of preventing small particles of dust and infectious matter from entering into the small air spaces where oxygenation of the blood takes place.

The lungs become less efficient as they clog with filth .... the mucus lining of the lungs becomes weakened and the whole body is starved of oxygen. Deprivation of oxygen to the brain can mean that the clear-thinking ability of a smoker is diminished by up to 23%. Smoking impairs your ability to concentrate .... it fogs your mind .. clouds your judgment .... but I don't want you to think about that too much.

Pulmonary emphysema .... chronic bronchitis .... lung cancer .... the coughs and the colds .... so frequent and so difficult to shake off .... the breathlessness that obliges you to use the lift when it would be so easy to use the stairs. The coughing .... the mucus .... the vile taste .... the awful smell now an integral part of you .... so offensive to those who object to your vile habit of smoking. You are intensely aware that you are not welcome in many public places .... theatres .... restaurants .... at work .... at play .... you indulge your habit out of sight .... in secret, ashamed, guilty. The taste and the smell that you have chosen for so long to ignore is now strong .... and from this moment forward you are reminded constantly .... powerfully .... in a manner which cannot be ignored each time that you are reminded of cigarettes.

Tissue which do not receive enough oxygen .... die .... as arteries become constricted and blocked .... arteriosclerosis becomes a word with particular meaning for you, as deprived of oxygen, ... part of you dies .... gangrene .... mortification of the flesh sets in .... and now, to save your life, a leg is surgically removed .... maybe both, or perhaps an arm. What is your quality of life now? Ask yourself right now and tell me clearly *(client's name)*; is this for you?

Heart disease .... stroke .... cancer of the liver .... the throat .... the pancreas .... the kidneys .... the tongue .... breast cancer .... cancer of the uterus .... of the ovaries .... of the testicles .... of the skin .... ulcers .... the list is endless and unforgiving, as the hospitals and modern medicine struggle to cope with the self-imposed destruction of those who are unwilling to accept the responsibility for their own life, their own health and happiness .... to protect and respect the miracle that is their own body.

***

It is a fact that the skin of a smoker ages more rapidly than that of a non-smoker. A fifty-year-old smoker is as old physically as a seventy-year-old non-smoker. Each cigarette reduces life expectancy by 6 minutes .... 20 per day means 2 hours of life that may never be .... but I don't want you to think about that too much.

The sexual prowess and potency of a smoker will diminish more rapidly with age than that of a non-smoker, and you can know that you can give so much more in that way by ensuring that you are fitter, more virile .... more attractive .... and that means non-smoker. Each smoker inhales just 15% of the smoke from their cigarette, the remainder goes directly into the atmosphere that we all have to breathe. Those whom you love and care for must also breathe the air that a smoker poisons. Perhaps you can agree with me that one very good reason for quitting this disgusting habit is that, through your excellent example, you may influence someone younger against taking up the habit. Just think of how much you could achieve, if just one young person was prevented from taking up the habit .... think of all the misery and the pain that could be prevented if that disgusting and costly mistake were avoided.

Now (*client's name*), please take a deep breath, and, as you release all of the air from your lungs, relax and go deeper .... as you allow your mind to show you yourself in a room .... all around you here are those you love and care for, and who love and care for you .... all who celebrate your decision to give up smoking and take the responsibility for your own health .... your own life .... to become your own person.

As you go deeper now, see them all before you, gathered here as you listen to the sound of my voice and the truth that is so important to you now. They are all here, they have come from far and near .... (*give names of significant people*) .... all have come because you have something to tell them .... a dreadful truth .... Your doctor has told you that you have contracted cancer and that you have but a short time to live, soon you will be gone .... You will be dead before your time, all because you ignored all the good advice, the wishes of those who wanted so much for you to give up smoking .... you made the choice .... a choice to die, and soon you will not be there for them who rely on you to be a part of their life.

You refused to accept the responsibility for your own health and for your own life, and now the immune system that you have relied on without consideration for so long to repair the ravages that you have inflicted upon your body, has given up .... overwhelmed .... defeated .... now you will die before your time and you must tell all here that terrible truth .... and tell them why .... and tell them who is responsible. Go ahead now and as you tell them, see their faces .... see the shock, the horror, the disbelief .... and then the anger .... the grief. And how do you feel?

An insidious habit has destroyed all .... your health, your life, wasted enormous amounts of money, enriching those few who would benefit without conscience or regard for the misery they purvey, selling in attractive packaging what you know to be no less than lethal poison.

Now feel the guilt .... the guilt that has for so long been repressed and ignored each time you lit up a cigarette .... Now feel it strongly .... so strong and powerful .... that feeling of shame when sneaking away to indulge in that filthy destructive habit away from friends and colleagues who are offended by it.

See ashtrays overflowing with stale and stinking cigarette butts .... burn holes in furnishings and in clothes..... stained paintwork and ceilings, brown and dingy..... intensely aware now of the smell that lingers and of the taste that disgusts you now each time you are reminded of cigarettes. And now remind yourself of your commitment, your promise to yourself .... that commitment now growing strong and powerful .... intense now .... your desire to pollute your mouth .... your body..... has gone completely .... and your subconscious mind helps you now with new and powerful responses and your desire to smoke has gone .... vanished completely, replaced with feelings of justifiable pride and deep personal satisfaction .... feelings of real and significant accomplishment.

Each day you feel stronger .... more alive .... your confidence and good feelings about yourself expand and grow .... become powerful .... no longer do you offend those about you with stinking tobacco-laden breath, stained teeth and reeking clothes and hair .... you are fitter, healthier, more attractive .... more alive.

As a non-smoker, you continue to enjoy a longer and healthier sex life and give so much more in that way. You experience pleasure that you are still capable of, long after the sexual prowess of a smoker of your age has failed them. No longer do you look for self- confidence .... for self-esteem .... for ways of coping with problems .... in packets of cigarettes .... You are aware that good feelings about yourself and your life come from deep within .... not from sticks of poisonous weed, false promises and illusions. There is no room for illusion in your life.

You see yourself now as a confident and self-assured non-smoker .... proud of your achievement .... those around you who continue to smoke do not concern you .... You wish for them the same good feelings and the freedom that you now experience .... the new- found reality that is life without the need or desire for the destructive effects of cigarettes. To them you express a gentle understanding indifference, coupled with your own firm resolve as you express and assert yourself always as that person who has no need or desire for cigarettes.

You can be intensely aware of the pride in your achievement each time you refuse cigarettes, and should you ever, through mistake or childish impulse, ever put a cigarette or tobacco product to your lips ever again ....

your subconscious mind will remind you in a powerful and unmistakable way .... of the nauseating smell, of the vile, disgusting taste, and of the guilt that attends each and every cigarette .... You will be reminded of your responsibility that cannot be passed to any other .... your health .... your life .... your body .... your commitment to yourself and those who love and care for you and who rely on you to be there.

***

Now you may decide to quit smoking right now .... or perhaps you may decide that later on today is a good time for you .... perhaps you may quit after lunch .... after dinner .... or just before you go to bed. Now I would prefer that you stop smoking immediately, but it's entirely up to you to discover .... today the right time for you to free yourself forever from smoking .... aware that your subconscious mind knows what to do for you, thinking with an awareness of things thought .... those things that are done automatically for you .... driving your car .... having no need or desire to smoke .... speaking on the telephone .... having no need or desire to smoke .... enjoying all those things that you have done before, and more, as that person who has lost any need or desire to smoke .... that person that now takes the full responsibility for life .... for health and happiness, and you can congratulate yourself right now on your excellent achievement, ... experience now the feeling of deep personal satisfaction as your confidence and your self-esteem grow and expand .... as your health and fitness improve with each and every new day .... that problem finally resolved.

***

And now as you feel so good about yourself, you can imagine that on a table in front of you now is a packet of those cigarettes that you used to smoke .... that you have wasted so much upon. Now see a strong wind blowing .... a powerful wind and see that wind blowing stronger and stronger .... blowing a gale now .... and see that powerful, cleansing wind scattering that packet of cigarettes and see the foul contents of the packet disintegrating and being swept away by that wind as it blows away each and every trace and every memory of that tobacco .... further .... further .... away into infinity, and with it every small desire to pollute your own body.

And when you can see that cleansing wind has done its work and all traces and memory of that tobacco have gone completely .... the wind drops and peace .... calm and tranquillity return completely now .... you see yourself clearly now as a natural non-smoker and you can tell me clearly .... "I am now a non-smoker".

(Wait for response)

That's good .... a very special part of you remembers clearly now the vile taste and the noxious odour of tobacco .... strong and intense .... and, should you ever through accident or childish, irresponsible impulse ever put a cigarette or tobacco product to your lips again, that part will provide you with an instant and disgusting reminder that you are a non-smoker .... responsible and proud. You are your own person.

Lifestyle Junction

You stopped smoking because you made a promise to yourself .... you made a commitment .... you made a decision .... but you know, it is more than that. What this all narrows down to is one very simple premise .... on this path of life you have been faced with a choice .... the choice that you are faced with is a junction on the road, a fork on the road of life, and a choice.

Of course you can continue down that same old road .... live your life with the smell, the cough, the phlegm and the colds that are so frequent and never seem to go away .... the shortness of breath, the guilt and the fear .... Of course you can continue living your life enslaved by packets of cigarettes .... or at this fork in the road .... this junction .... you can choose to turn off the beaten track .... to take that turning off to the right .... onto a new road of opportunity .... to continue living your life in a new and powerfully positive and exciting way .... healthy .... strong .... vital .... vibrant .... powerfully alive and free from the bonds and chains that are cigarettes .... You are at that fork in the road right now .... now you must make that choice, and I want you to tell me which road do you intend to take from here?

(Pause for reply)

Now tell me what that road looks like .... what do you see?

Repeat and affirm client's description of the road, emphasizing the cleanness and the freshness of the air, the perfume of flowers and the taste of food, fitness and health etc., etc.

Affirmation Of Inner Self

This script can be used at any time to allow the client the opportunity to experience something pleasant and positive.

And now, as you allow that trance to continue and to deepen even more, I wonder how much more comfortable and tranquil you really can become .... aware now perhaps of that pleasant heaviness of arms .... of legs .... of the whole body, that just seems to be there but then perhaps some way off from here .... there in that chair resting .... comfortable .... while the conscious mind continues to drift and allow the subconscious more and more of the responsibility for allowing that awareness of just how little you need to concern yourself about things that are of little moment.

It can happen if you wish .... that your subconscious mind can allow you an opportunity to experience those things which are pleasant and positive .... to surprise you perhaps with a pleasant thought .... a long forgotten memory of a happy event .... even a taste or a fragrance .... a warm and all-embracing feeling of being at one with yourself .... a brilliant colour that will suddenly evoke that feeling .... that memory .... that pleasant feeling of how wonderful it is to be alive to experience those moments that really do stand out .... wonderful times of pleasant experience .... and you can know then that you really do not need to know just how your subconscious mind knows how to do that for you in that way .... simply take the moment, and bask in the light of that revelation .... as your subconscious mind opens up .... allowing that inner voice and that creative and unique part of you to give to you that gift .... that feeling that will allow you to understand even more.

Weight On The Mind

One of the problems which so many people present to a hypnotherapist is that of weight. Of course, there are so many considerations to take into account when dealing with these unhappy people who feel so bad about themselves.

Overeating is so often just a symptom of the underlying problem, and the phrase "weight on the mind" can seem so very appropriate.

For the person who is overweight, the problem of self-image is extremely acute, and it can be argued that the dictates of fashion can be a powerful factor in shaping the image of self which is so important and so powerful.

We need to ask why this person is compelled to overeat when it really does make him/her miserable. Can it be that they wish to make themselves unattractive to the opposite sex in order to avoid having to form relationships?

Is the food eaten as a substitute for love and affection missing in that person's life? Perhaps it is just a habit by the manner in which the parents encouraged the child to eat up everything on the plate. "Eat it all up now. Think of all the starving children in Africa"; powerful incantations that can stay with us into adult life. Isn't this logic a little strange though, that, by eating much more food than we actually need, we can compensate for the fact of another's hunger? The concept of waste can be a powerful factor. For many of us, our parents will have experienced times of shortage and hardship which in these modern times cannot really be appreciated. The message "waste not, want not" is passed through the generations, and the habit passed on from parent to child. I have a new message which I consider much more appropriate and effective: "You can waste food in the bin, or you can waste it on your waist .... waste to waist."

It is important that the therapist considers carefully the course of intervention that will be used to help the overweight client. Investigate thoroughly the background of the client, and if necessary use analysis to determine the true motivations before wading in with suggestion therapy which could prove inappropriate.

Personally, I favour an approach using the "six-step reframe" at the first appointment, and then gauging the response of the client during the following week. At the second appointment, it will be easier to determine the course that the therapy should then take. The fact is, there is no easy answer that will apply in all cases.

Each one will be different, and must be treated in a manner which is well-considered.

The scripts provided for weight therapy should always be used taking account of the person, and only the therapist can make the decision as to the advisability of a particular approach.

Weight – What I Tell 'Em

The following paragraphs are a condensation of the talks that I give to groups of people who are interested in losing weight. I include it, because I believe that it helps to be able to speak to clients with some authority, thereby gaining their confidence. You may disagree with some of the content. That's fine. Wouldn't it be a dreary old world if nobody questioned or put forward new thoughts and ideas? In this profession, the discussion of old and new ideas and strategies can only help us all to be the best therapists that we can, and in that way we serve those who need us to the best of our ability.

Eating For Life

We all have to eat. Marvellous as our bodies are, they are in fact very complex machines which require fuel in order to function. We require energy in order to be active and, in the same way a car burns either petrol or diesel as fuel, we 'burn' food.

When our car is burning too much fuel, how quick we are to tackle the problem. After all, it costs money to fill the tank. Excessive fuel consumption means that the engine is consuming too much for the amount of power that it returns, and so down goes the M.P.G.. The excess fuel cannot be burned efficiently, and so it ends up as thick carbon deposits which gum up the works and reduce the effectiveness of the engine. The life of the engine will be reduced if the problem is not attended to quickly.

In the same way, if we overload our engine with more food than it needs and/or use the wrong types of fuel, then our performance will be affected. We will build up deposits of unburned fuel in the form of body fat and, of course, the efficiency and the life expectancy will be reduced as we place extra loading upon it.

I have no intention of laying out a specific and rigid diet. In all probability, you will have tried most of the clever diets; the exotic and different ways of losing excess pounds, and by now you will have realized that the only thing you will lose permanently is money paid out for the marvellous products which you feed yourself with in order to lose weight. What I will outline for you is a basis on which you can take control of your own eating habits and the responsibility for your own health and well-being.

First we have to address our eating habits and be honest with ourselves. When do we eat, where do we eat and how do we eat? Why do we eat?

Do you chew your food thoroughly, savouring each mouthful, or make a race of it, cramming in as much as possible in a short time?

Do you eat on the run? Do you reward yourself with food? Do you pacify yourself, in times of trouble and stress, with food? Do you eat snacks between your main meals? Do you reward your children with food? Do you give your children a snack so that you too can enjoy a treat?

An extremely important question that you must ask yourself is: "Do I really want to lose weight?", and if the answer is "Yes", then "Why?" Make sure that what you are doing is for you and your self-esteem and not a fad of convention. You should be happy with yourself and your decisions.

Okay, now we get down to a plan of action that is going to achieve what you want for yourself. Set yourself attainable goals and believe always that you can and you will do this for yourself. First I want you to take a good look at when you eat and where you eat. If you do not eat at set times during the day, then right now resolve to eat at a time which you will designate as a mealtime. Make it a mealtime for all the family as much as is possible.

Where do you eat? If you find yourself, as so many do these days, sitting down in front of the television with a tray upon your lap, then I want you never to do that again. Eat at the table and, when you eat, concentrate on what you are doing. You do not eat while doing other things. You now eat slowly, chew your food properly and savour the taste and the texture, amazed at how much more enjoyment you will get from mealtimes if you take the time to taste your food.

When you feel hunger, what in fact is happening is that a tiny sensor at the base of the brain, called the hypothalamus, is sending a message to let you know that it is time to eat. About 20 minutes after it has told you that you need to eat, it then sends another message telling you that it is satisfied, and the feelings associated with hunger subside. Just think now of all the times when you felt hungry and, even though you did not eat, the hunger pangs just went away. This is important for you to know, because from this moment forward you are aware that it is not how much you eat during that twenty minutes that will satisfy the feelings of hunger at all. The hypothalamus will allow you to eat as much or as little as possible in that twenty minutes before sending the exact same message of satisfaction. Crazy but true!

As you begin to lose weight, it will be necessary for you to drink plenty. It doesn't matter too much what you drink, as long as it is not alcohol, which has much in the way of calories but next to nought in the way of nutrition. Drinks with high sugar content must be avoided. If you decide that you can stick to mineral or spa water then that is fine, as is tea and coffee without sugar. The more you drink, the more you will need to go to the bathroom and in a very natural manner flush away the toxins that are stored in the body fats.

Now for some of the more serious don'ts: there are of course foods which are extremely non-beneficial in our quest for the slim and attractive body that is hidden within those extra pounds. White flour products are definitely bad news: these include cakes and pies, white bread, biscuits, sausage rolls and so on. White, refined flour. Burn this now into your mind and resolve to ensure that you will ever be on your guard to ensure that you do not buy or bake foods with white, refined flour. Bread made with wholemeal flour is fine, and will prove a very potent weapon in your fight to retain the slim and elegant you that you are going to be. Make a list of all of the white flour products that you can think of. Now have a look in your cupboards to see how many of these products are lurking there. Now do the same for products made with wholemeal flour and see how much real choice you have in designing a healthy eating regime for yourself.

Many dairy products are to be avoided. Think now of the contents of the dairy cabinet at your supermarket and you will find it easy, with just a little care, to determine which of those products have a lower fat content. Low-fat spreads and cheeses, yoghurts and many other treats can be found with low fat contents. Why, they even make low-fat ice cream these days. It will surprise you, too, how the once mundane task of getting in the weekly shopping can now prove to be an interesting experience. You will enjoy the quest for those foods which are healthy and beneficial, and surprise, surprise, the tills will not ring so loudly either.

No longer will you experience that pang of guilt, when you choose those foods which you know are not part of your healthy eating plan. Being slim will improve your love-life! There, that grabbed your attention, did it not? If you feel more attractive, then you will project that feeling in your love-making, and that can be much more exciting that munching on a cream bun. Am I right?

As you begin to lose the weight that has been with you for so long, you will feel better about yourself, more confident and more energetic, no longer having to carry around with you that excess fat. As you feel better, you will become more determined to increase that feeling of well-being, more motivated to become the person who is in control, who has the body that you want and that you deserve.

Fruit and vegetables become a regular part of your daily diet. Why not ensure that there is fruit, celery and carrot, etc, in the fridge, cut up into snack sized pieces? Do not allow yourself to become obsessed with foods that you cannot have. It does not pay to be too hard on yourself and, if you do make a slip, just accept that you are human and then carry on with your eating plan. Do not treat any food as taboo. You are fully aware of what is good and what is not, and you are also aware of whose responsibility it is to look after your body and of how good you feel as you move ever closer to your goal.

Diamond Weight Control

First (*client's name*), I would like you to know how much I appreciate and admire you for the decision that you have taken, to take on for yourself fully the responsibility for your own life .... to respect and protect your own body.

It is with our body that we enjoy the good things of life ... and today you decided that it is time to take the action that you need to take .... to change those ways of doing things in that way .... the right way for you.

You are aware of your desire to eat good food .... you are aware that your body needs food to remain healthy .... and you are also aware that there are foods which are good and nutritious, and that there are foods which can do you harm .... make you fat ... making you feel sad .... feel very guilty and then very angry .... and then these negative emotions harm you also.

Now that you have taken your decision to lose weight .... and to respect your own body .... you will be pleasantly surprised at how easily you will be able to achieve your goal .... a slim and healthy, attractive body.

I wonder if you can imagine, just how many people come here to ask me for help with this problem or that .... who will tell me that they do not have the drive or the determination to succeed .... to make those changes for themselves which are necessary to improve the quality of their life. ....

I tell all of those people .... the person who has no drive, did not make an appointment .... that person who has no determination did not arrive on time if at all .... and that person who has no vision is not sitting there in that chair so relaxed and so comfortable .... you have all that you need to do all of those things and to achieve your worthwhile goals .... but there is just one thing that you do not have, that you will take with you when you leave here today .... that is confidence .... confidence that you recognise now .... of the kind it takes to tackle any task .... or set out on a journey knowing that you have done all that is required .... made all arrangements .... certain that you will complete the task or journey safely .... quickly and without fuss .... just as you recognise now those signs of success in achieving a wonderfully relaxed and comfortable state .... sensing a gentle connection with your perfect inner self that tells you that you can .... you will .... that you have all of the confidence that you need .... recognising too those heavy, comfortable feelings as your whole body relaxes and your mind relaxes deeper and deeper with each word that I speak.

I am reminded now of a man who built himself a fine house .... a house that he designed himself .... built on a plot of land right on the edge of town, with fantastic views over rolling hills and valleys to the sea. He had a dream of building this house for many years and spent so many long hours poring over the drawings .... imagining himself in that house .... enjoying the garden .... the pool .... planning how he would furnish it and decorate it. Then came the day when his hard work and his planning came to fruition .... and he bought the plot of land .... and he built that house just as he dreamed it .... furnished it .... decorated it exactly how he wanted it. He married his true love, and I wonder if you can know how proud he felt as he carried his new bride over the threshold of that dream home. He spent many hours in that house .... for he worked from home in an office that he had incorporated in the plans ..... and as he worked, his new wife busied herself around the house in the way that a wife does to make a house a home. .... Neither of them noticed at first the feelings of lethargy .... the constant headaches that never seemed to ease ..... putting it down to working too hard at ensuring that their home and their life was as perfect as could be. They consulted their doctor and he gave them pills and potions, but to no avail .... they never seemed to feel any better .... feeling that their health was just fading away .... but they did have a beautiful home. It was over two years before they got round to taking a holiday .... jetting off to the delights of foreign lands .... and they were both amazed, that after just a few days .... all the feelings of lethargy ..... the headaches .... just disappeared: .... they were their old selves once again.

On their return .... the husband made some enquiries .... speaking to some of the local farmers, and was amazed to discover that the land he had built his house upon was contaminated .... an old dumping ground .... He called in an expert and was told that poisonous chemicals were present in the soil .... and gases were seeping from the ground poisoning his house and poisoning both him and his wife. It took just a day for him to get out of that house .... for he knew that his health and that of those he loved were more important than any house .... no matter how much he had wanted it.

Nobody likes to be told what to do .... and if I were able to tell you what to do .... then you would have no need at all to be here today .... you would simply call me on the 'phone and say .... "(therapist's name), I would like to lose weight and be able to wear the clothes that I would like to wear .... in a size .... (desired dress size)," .... and I would say to you ...."(client's name), ... that's a great idea .... stop overeating and eating those foods that are unhealthy and fattening and instead eat only those foods which are healthy and non-fattening .... do it right now." .... But nobody likes to be told what to do .... so I wouldn't say to you that overeating and eating those foods which are unhealthy and which make you fat .... are dangerous .... They are dangerous and will prevent you from having the body that you desire .... the body that you are entitled to .... the body that you deserve .... slim and firm and beautiful .... and I needn't tell you that you will get no pleasure from butter and cheese .... or from any dairy products that are so high in fat content and so high in calories .... fattening and unhealthy foods .... you will get no pleasure from overeating .... but you will become aware of feelings of great pride and accomplishment when you choose foods that are healthy and non-fattening. I need never say to you that overeating .... unhealthy and fattening foods is no substitute for lack of adequate stimulation in your life .... or for love that you need and are entitled to have .... I need never tell you that you do not need to eat more food than is necessary to maintain your body at the weight that will allow you to wear the clothes that you choose in a size (*desired dress size*) .... weighing a comfortable slim and lovely .... (*target weight*). But one thing I will say to you .... is that controlling your eating is not something that you will not find easy .... and when you leave here today you will no longer be that person who overeats and eats those foods which are unhealthy and fattening ..... you know that you have a desire for foods like biscuits .... butter .... cheese .... cakes .... sweet things with lots of sugar .... and you know that nobody can talk you out of it .... But what you know now .... that you didn't before .... is that you also have an enormous amount of NO DESIRE .... and you can get to know this place of ... NO DESIRE .... as it expands and reaches deeper and deeper and the feelings of .... NO DESIRE .... can reach even deeper .... and the time of .... NO DESIRE .... grow longer and longer .... and no way is easier than this.

That house was a lovely dream, but the price was just too much to pay .... and it's good to finally resolve those feelings and to just let go .... not needing to know how the unconscious mind knows what to do for you .... thinking with an awareness of things .... thoughts .... without the need to know those things that are done automatically .... You know what to do .... now I would prefer that you stop overeating .... and eating unhealthy and fattening foods right away .... immediately .... but it's entirely up to you to discover the time .... today .... the best time and the best way for you .... some people wait an hour .... some wait until they have used up stocks of food at home .... and then some stop entirely before they go to bed .... Now I'd prefer that you stop right now .... immediately .... but it's entirely up to you to choose a time today when you free yourself forever from this unhealthy and fattening habit forever.

We have all suffered the loss of some one that we love .... or something or situation that we value .... and we can be aware that gone is an important part of our life.

You can be aware right now of the responsibility that you have towards those who love you and care for you .... who you love and care for .... special people who rely on you to be there for them .... the responsibility that is yours and yours alone to ensure that those people will not be faced with the loss of that person .... whom they love and treasure .... responsibility to ensure that you live a healthy and long life .... respecting and protecting your body .... cherishing your gift of life .... that person eating just what you need .... eating foods which are healthy and in the right amounts and at the right times.

You can waste food .... you can waste it .... put it into the bin .... or you can waste food on your waist .... waste to waist .... I wonder what you will prefer. Whenever you see those foods which are unhealthy .... foods which will pile on the pounds .... you will be reminded in a manner that is instant and powerful as your subconscious mind helps you .... reminds you of your commitment with images of you that have distressed you and those feelings of guilt and sadness that attend that fat, overweight person that you used to be. You accept now without reservation the total responsibility for your own health .... your own life .... your own happiness .... You are now your own person .... proud and confident .... You see yourself always as that person in control of her life .... slim, lithe and lovely .... that problem finally resolved.

(Go to trance termination)

"Swish Pattern" Weight Loss

First, establish with your client the weight he/she wishes to be, dress size etc.

Establish goals. Establish that the subconscious is very specific and that, if the goal is a realistic one, then it will happen.

Diets: Deprivation .... the basic instinct of the subconscious is survival, and deprivation does not fit in with that concept. Comfortable, however, does fit .... it's nice to be comfortable.

Imagine now that you are in a restaurant watching some slim people looking through the menu. What are they doing? .... mentally they are tasting the food .... visualizing how it will look served on the plate .... what they are not thinking about is how comfortable they will feel .... food remains in the stomach for up to four hours and it is important to know how comfortable that will feel.

Now what I want you to be thinking about is yourself .... *(desired weight loss)* .... think about how good you will feel about yourself .... how good you will look .... what you are wearing .... and what your friends and family will think about how good you look .... but I don't want you to think about that too much.

Now we will do some hypnosis and during the course of this therapy which is all for your benefit and, only with your approval, I will need at times to touch your hands .... your forehead .... and then your knee .... I'm telling you this so there is no reason for you to be surprised, and my touch will relax you deeper. Just visualize how you will feel .... lighter .... just how does that feel?
Induction for hypnosis ....

Now *(client's name)*, I want you to go to a special and very pleasant memory of yours .... in the past .... a memory of importance .... of significance to you. There may be a few, but your subconscious mind will understand and know exactly which one is of importance to you now .... of significance to you now .... and unconsciously you know it is of value to you now .... you know as it selects itself .... as you experience those successful feelings .... of importance .... of significance to you now. For you know that the answers come from that memory held way back then. And now go deeper and as you drift down deeper and deeper now .... I know that I really don't have to tell you that the deeper, you go the better you feel .... and the better you feel, the deeper you go.

And now in your mind .... in your imagination .... I want you to go to a special room .... a special room of belief and of capability .... in this room you will see that there is only one piece of furniture .... that is a television set .... now you can speak to me but you cannot wake .... when you see it .... just say "yes".

That's good .... now what I would like you to do is to put onto the blank screen of that television .... all of that extra weight that you have .... that you want to lose .... put it all up there on that screen .... all of those extra fat cells .... perhaps you can see them as pinkish in colour .... perhaps orangey .... all piled up as a fatty mass .... Now put into the picture just how uncomfortable you feel when you overeat .... Now put into the picture what your family and friends think when you overeat .... now all of the reasons that you have for your need to overeat .... be it lack of love .... unhappiness .... whatever those reasons your subconscious mind knows exactly what is meant here .... just put it all there on that screen. Now put onto that screen all of the damage that overeating does .... all that cholesterol .... high blood pressure .... breathlessness .... the danger of heart attack and stroke .... that uncomfortable feeling when you overeat and also that feeling of guilt and of shame .... shame that you are not taking on the responsibility for your own health and well being .... carrying all of that extra weight .... When you have that picture really clearly in your mind say "yes". *(When the client says "yes" continue.)* .... I now want you to store this picture somewhere convenient in your mind because we will need it later ....

Okay *(client's name)* .... that's good .... now I want you to see another picture there on that screen .... a smaller, inset picture in the top right of the screen .... make this picture one of *(client's name)* now having lost that extra weight *(target weight loss)*, lighter in a dress size *(target size)* .... notice how good she feels .... how she looks .... that feeling of confidence .... increased self-esteem .... happier .... more alive .... lighter in all ways .... *(client's name)* taking care of herself .... and with that feeling of huge optimism.

Now I want you to give *(client's name)* in this picture, on a scale of one to ten .... for confidence .... ten .... for self-esteem .... ten .... give her a score of ten for self-respect.

This is the *(client's name)* who eats only when her appetite says she is hungry .... the *(client's name)* who stops eating when her appetite tells that it is right .... a friend of her appetite .... who is aware that on her tongue are 26,000 taste buds, and when she puts food into her mouth they will very quickly become satisfied .... who chews her food slowly and thoroughly and carefully until her appetite is satisfied .... the *(client's name)* who is fully aware that any more food than is enough to satisfy her appetite .... is waste .... and that waste can either be wasted in the bin .... or wasted on her waist .... waste to waist.

Now in a moment as you watch the screen .... you will hear me say the word "Swish" .... and you can make that small picture grow .... spread across the screen .... that picture of the new you. You will do this very fast and you will do this five time as this is how the subconscious learns .... "SWISH" .... erasing all of those old eating habits .... SWISHING .... erasing all of that extra weight .... all of that discomfort .... that feeling of guilt .... of shame .... until that picture fills the screen eliminating completely that old picture .... filling the screen with that new *(client's name)*.

Now make the screen go blank and put back the old picture and notice what is different about it .... put back the inset picture in the top right corner of the screen .... and now "SWISH" .... again .... "SWISHING" .... erasing .... that old *(client's name)* .... eliminating that excess weight .... "SWISHING" erasing all of those feeling of discomfort .... of lack of confidence .... eliminating those feelings of guilt .... all of those bad eating habits .... all of those negative feelings erased and eliminated as the new *(client's name)* fills the screen completely now.

Now make the screen go blank .... put back the old picture on the screen .... notice what's different .... look at the colour now and tell me what is different about that picture.

(Give client time to tell you what is different .... and then ....)

Now .... "SWISH" again .... *(repeat sequence)*

Now walk over to that television set and turn up the colour .... turn it up as high as it will go .... Now "SWISH" again .... *(repeat sequence)*

Now make the screen go blank .... and put on it now all that remains of that old picture .... the small remains .... the dregs of that old picture .... the smallest traces .... and then "SWISH" again .... erasing all that remains of that old picture .... all that remains of those old eating habits .... those bad feelings .... eliminating completely all of that extra weight .... those feelings of discomfort .... as the new and exciting *(client's name)* fills the screen completely now .... see the new and so confident *(client's name)* .... lighter *(client's name)* .... filling that screen completely now in full and glorious colour .... And now let those wonderful feelings expand and grow now .... *(Anchor good feelings .... touch knee with firm pressure for approximately 10 to 15 seconds.)*

Now step into that picture .... into that TV set, and try out that new body .... that slim and lovely *(client's name)* .... *(desired weight loss)* lighter .... striding out now happy .... smiling .... looking absolutely wonderful .... wearing a beautiful new dress .... size *(target size)* .... walk about now and experience fully that comfort .... that confidence, that self-esteem .... proud now .... slim and attractive ....lithe and lovely .... enjoy that experience and become familiar with the new *(client's name)*.

Now go forward in time .... *(client's name)*, ... *(target loss)* lighter .... wearing that dress in a size *(target size)* .... now a date will flash as your subconscious chooses one that is significant and appropriate .... tell me what is that date? Are you satisfied with that date .... you will be happy to be *(target weight loss)* lighter on .... *(date given)*.

Okay .... now *(client's name)* .... please take a deep breath and go deep inside and try .... try in vain to have that same problem .... It was a terrible problem wasn't it? .... You want to make those changes about you .... think about those changes now .... in the future as you look back and think about it now .... to make that change now for yourself, so that you could stop having that problem now and see yourself now.

Do you like the way that you look? Just look back at yourself having made that change now .... and you will, will you not?

"Swish Pattern" originated by Richard Bandler, 1982

Physical Dissociation

And when your thoughts begin to travel faster than your body can keep up with .... you can re-discover how the mind can travel so far and so fast .... and you can wonder about things that exist in the universe .... the size of the mighty ocean .... the age of the huge trees that fill the sky .... and the number of stars in the night sky .... things that you have wondered about from time to time .... and you can let your mind float freely in that place that you find yourself drawn to .... while your body remains here .... comfortably here .... there is no need to disturb it .... no need to allow it to hold you back .... You can just enjoy the freedom of letting your mind float freely .... to the places that you most enjoy .... and while your mind is there .... and your body is here .... it can be so comforting to know that your body is here .... waiting comfortably .... patiently for as long as you'd like it to float freely without having to notice it .... because your mind can go anywhere that it wants to go.

Amnesia

And as your mind continues to relax .... each breath soothing you .... I wonder how much attention you have paid to the different thoughts floating through your mind .... Your mind can be so active as it relaxes .... and then you can realise how difficult it is to remember .... what I was talking about exactly seven minutes ago .... and you could try to remember what I was saying nine minutes ago .... or what you were thinking four minutes ago .... but doesn't it seem like just too much work .... to try to remember .... it takes more effort than it's worth .... so much easier to allow yourself to relax comfortably .... knowing that you don't have to remember when it really is too much work .... too much effort to bother making ....

Confusion Technique
To Facilitate Amnesia

And now that you have had the opportunity to discover new possibilities .... while you can learn from past experiences .... your conscious mind can begin to wonder how it will know which things to remember .... and which things only your subconscious need know .... and then you can remember to forget .... or you may choose to forget to remember .... Your memory of forgetting forgets what it has forgotten .... but you can only forget what you have forgotten when you realise it's too difficult to remember anyway .... and then you can forget all the confusion .... and relax even more deeply than before ....

Coping With Abreaction

When a client experiences the emotions that are attached to long- repressed memories, the event can be extremely dramatic and to a degree quite daunting for the therapist. The importance of the therapist's remaining calm and reassuring is paramount as he/she continues to speak to the client in a voice which is calming and confident.

Explain to the client that the event being experienced is of importance and that there is no need to fear it, as it is but a memory. Initially it was frightening but, having survived the original event, there is no question of its having any power to harm ever again. Now, in the light of conscious awareness, it has lost entirely its power to hurt.

Before initiating a regression session with a client, I make a provision, for example, of suggesting that, if I place my hand on his/her forehead, then he/she will immediately return to the place of safety that has been provided before the regression. This can be a garden, or a beach, a familiar room, etc.. It matters not, as long as it is a place where the client can feel safe and secure.

Having calmed the situation and restored the client to a relaxed state, I will then invite the client to return to the same scenario which frightened him/her so much. The difference, however, is that first I explain the importance of reviewing the event in order that it can be finally resolved, and a more beneficial perspective formed.

The use of visualization can include dissociative techniques - perhaps a video of the event, suggesting to the client that he/she has a remote control with which the video can be run, stopped, backed up, freeze-framed or run forward. The more control that can be suggested, the more comfortable the client will feel, and in this way he/she will feel in control over the past problem area.

Approach the situation by degrees, perhaps allowing just the sound of someone speaking about the event, or perhaps looking at the scene from far away. As he/she draws nearer, the event can be run through without the client actually in the picture at first, then little by little the scene can be added to at a comfortable pace, including the introduction of the client into the scenario.

"And now that you do know what is really occurring there .... you are able to see yourself very clearly in that place at that time .... on the count of three you will be there at that place and at that time".

There are so many ways that this situation can be approached, limited only by the imagination and expertise of the therapist. You will be there to determine how you will need to tailor your approach in a professional and reassuring manner.

"I know and you know too that this event at this time and place is very important and significant to you .... and I would like you to take me along with you as you re-experience now the whole event .... but because I am not able to see or hear what is happening .... or know about your feelings and emotions .... please help me by telling me what is happening .... and how you are feeling .... there is nothing here that can harm you and I want you to know that I am with you here and you are quite safe".

Calm is the key, with the understanding that no harm can come to your client here as he/she releases what is after all emotion that has been contained harmfully for so long. The abreaction is a release and to you, the therapist, the most potent indicator that significant progress is occurring. A large box of man-sized tissues is a must for every consulting room.

Audio & Videotape Therapy

I expect that I am one among many who use pre-recorded audiotapes with my clients. I consider that they are useful in compounding and reinforcing the content of therapeutic sessions, but would question their value without the planned and considered intervention tailored individually to each client.

I would certainly raise an eyebrow at some therapists' use of taped inductions and suggestion therapy sessions. My argument in this case would be that each and every client is unique, and the valuable and personal utilization of events during the induction and therapy will be lost as the opportunity is missed. "And as you clear your throat, I wonder if you can notice how much more comfortable you become now with each breath that you take," *and* "You can hear the telephone ringing now, and know that it does not concern you; each ring is but a signal for you to go deeper still."

I explain to my clients that the tapes that I supply are to reinforce what happens in the consulting room and that they will most certainly help, provided that the instructions I give are followed in their use. The suggestion, "If you do this, you will be helped", *is obviously important as it affirms to the client that listening to the tapes will be of value and so he/she will benefit.*

Providing a client with a tape is in effect "compounding". "As you listen to the tape you will become aware of a new confidence." *In the same way, we suggest to a client,* "As your left arm grows heavier, then so the right arm will become lighter and you may be aware of how heavy that heavy arm is now". *It is all suggestion and acceptance by the client.*

Much has been said by others more learned than me, certainly more willing to express their views and expose them to public scrutiny, regarding the "placebo" effect. The fact that we, as therapists, do what we do by suggestion and are effective through the compliance of our clients would suggest that the placebo element is not to be denied. In my engineering days, there was a generally accepted premise: "If it's not broke, don't fix it." *I would suggest that this can be reasonably applied to any arguments that follow this direction.*

Providing a person with a "medicine" that is nothing more than perhaps a sugar solution and telling them with authority, "Drink this and you will feel better", *can easily be equated with suggestion therapy. Placebo maybe, but what the hell? If it works, if it proves beneficial to those who come to us seeking help, then call it what you will, but use it and you will experience the gratitude of those who, maybe because they have believed that they will be helped, are helped. Therefore you have helped them, and do not need to justify something of whose immense value you are confident.*

When making tapes, the option of having music playing softly in the background can seem an attractive proposition but I have moved away from this. My attitude to making tapes is that I wish, not so much to produce a commercially viable product, as to provide for my clients the best content of most benefit to them. A tape is purely therapeutic and specially formulated, first to relax through the use of an hypnotic induction, and then to deliver positive affirmations and suggestions to the subconscious during the relaxed state thus induced.

I remember clearly being informed by a client that she had not listened more than once to the tape which I had supplied to her, as she found the music annoying. My reply: "That's interesting: did you feel perhaps that you needed to be entertained?" Obviously there are other messages within the statement, but let us not get too embroiled!

Music, however, can provide a useful vehicle within which to embed subliminal messages, and the tapes which I supply have on one side exactly that utilization, the advantage being that the tape can then be listened to at any time without danger, as long as it is the subliminal side and not the therapy side that is playing whilst driving the car.

Subliminal messages embedded within music are effective in that they by-pass completely the critical analytical processes of the conscious mind and deliver, unaltered by perception, those messages to the subconscious. This negation of the conscious mind to rationalize the content is extremely effective, and provides a powerful medium for therapeutic change.

I have heard the term "brain-washing" used by some. Well, I do not wish to become embroiled in any argument. The active content contained in the messages will help provide those changes which are desirable for the client, so I fail to see where any cause for complaint can arise.

Tapes should always carry a specific warning regarding their use and, in particular, the side that carries an hypnotic induction should never be used whilst driving or operating machinery. The dangers are obvious to those who are aware, but perhaps, just perhaps, there may be someone who is not aware and who could end up wrapped around a motorway bridge pillar as a result, so we must warn clients. Personally, I do so both by way of written instructions on how to use the tape, and then verbally at the start, before the induction.

In recent years, the development of video technology and the fact that now most homes do have a video player has resulted in the introduction of therapeutic video programmes using strategies hitherto unavailable to therapists.

I have seen a number of these videos, some of them utter rubbish and some, well, they do have some merit. But I am mindful of the powerful therapeutic qualities that are found utilized in the medium of "psychovisual therapy". This system was developed by a young graphics designer who combined his skills in computers and video technology to produce a series of unique video programmes.

The first of these was simply named "Relaxation", and used a mixture of colours (chromotherapy) and changing shapes, combined with music and subliminal messages, literally to bombard the viewer with relaxation cues, so that a light trance would be induced.

"As a hypnoanalyst myself, I immediately recognized the potential in PsyV, not just as a technique for relaxation but as a valuable aid in therapy."

Michael Carr-Jones, 1992

The popularity of the first title soon resulted in other titles, and before too long a small library was available. "Stop Smoking" was produced with the co-operation of a number of experts in the fields of hypnotherapy, art and music. While the viewer watched the beautiful undulating shapes and colours, listening to the soothing relaxing music, a state of light hypnosis was induced and, whilst the viewer was relaxed and open to suggestion, the therapy content provided powerful positive messages to promote beneficial change and reduction of the desire to smoke.

The success rate of the use of this programme in conjunction with traditional hypnotherapy proved very encouraging. Of the group comprising the trial subjects, in excess of 90% were still not smoking after six months.

Originally I began "Stop Smoking" therapy by conducting a standard hypnotherapy session with my clients and then, following trance termination, would have them view the programme through in my office, before having them take the video home to continue the therapy. I was following the recommended format for using PsyV, but I soon began to question the order of march, and then elected to turn the whole thing about.

I proceed by carrying out the initial information-gathering exercise and then directly to having the client view the programme; after all, the video contained an hypnotic induction, and my task proved so much easier when the time came formally to induce eyes-closed hypnosis.

The client, having purchased a copy of the video, takes it home, with my instructions that it be viewed at least once a day for the next seven to ten days, then at regular intervals, and finally as and when the need arises.

My success rate has proved very good, and, while not being in a position to quote scientifically-derived figures, I would not feel too ambitious in my claim of around 90% success.

The psychovisual titles are now marketed in this country by Psychovisual Libraries of Poole in Dorset, the company formed some ten years ago by Michael Carr-Jones, himself a well-respected hypnotherapist in his own right.

The videos are not sold directly to the public, but through approved clinics and health professionals. Many medical facilities have used, to good effect, the range of titles available, recognizing their potential for providing a valuable aid in therapy. They gently create new and positive images to lift the self-esteem, forming new and beneficial habit patterns when the new values and positive motivations are stored as the imagination is stimulated to create personal positivity, confidence and well-being, to be held in memory.

It is a fact that the "Stop Smoking" PsyV programme is the only therapeutic video to have received the accolade of acceptance from the British Medical Association, in recognition of its value as a therapeutic medium. It has also received a prestigious B.L.A.T. award from the British Life Assurance Trust.

More information about Psychovisual Therapy can be obtained by writing to:

Lifestyle Libraries,
PO Box 1193,
POOLE,
Dorset. BH14 8YT
United Kingdom.

Internet Address: Psychovisual@compuserve.com

Hypnosis In Entertainment

"There is, I know, a growing strength of feeling within the profession regarding the use of hypnosis for entertainment purposes. I am not alone in my misgivings at what can be a demeaning of something which is, after all, a proven, effective therapeutic tool.

"Many people will not seek out hypnosis as a therapeutic alternative as a result of having watched stage hypnotism, because they cannot even begin to comprehend how what they have seen in a night club show can be used clinically to help someone in distress.

"Colleagues of mine have pointed out that many people seek out hypnosis in therapy because of the stage hypnotist, but such people tend to believe that hypnotists have mysterious powers, and so they approach treatment unrealistically."

Michael Yapko, 1990.

There is a danger, of course, that the imagination, unfettered by the critical, analytical conscious mind, will allow emotions and images to be created which will be accepted in memory as if in actuality.

Certain sensations and effects can be suggested which are potentially dangerous: in the same way that the power of suggestion can be used to help someone to stop smoking or biting their nails, suggestions can also, if delivered in an untrained and irresponsible way, promote a behavioural or emotional response not intended.

For those who have undergone formal training, the phrase "symptom substitution" will go some way towards the emphasis I seek here. As a therapist, I am aware that when I facilitate the removal of a symptomatic response, I must take care to ensure that I have dealt with the causative event, to ensure that I have not just made way for another, equally detrimental, substitute symptomatic response.

When using "Parts Therapy", it always good practice to instruct the "part" which is responsible for the symptom to accept a new and more beneficial task, an implanted substitute, such as helping with confidence or in a particular circumstance.

There are so many incidents where harm is done when an untrained and, dare I say, irresponsible person begins to make fun, tinkering with the delicate intricacies of the human psyche.

I paid a lot of money for my car; it represents, to me, a major investment. When I take it for its regular servicing or for repair, I am content that the garage which I have used for many years is equipped with all the necessary tools, and that the technician who will tend to my pride and joy is properly trained and is qualified to do the work. I certainly would not entrust my car to an untrained and unqualified jerk whose only tool was a rather large hammer.

It seems reasonable that, when dealing with something as complex as the human psyche, we should ensure that unqualified thrill- seekers are not let loose with nothing more than the "large hammer" which equates so well with an easily-learned ability to induce hypnosis in very susceptible people.

It is necessary to look very carefully at the use of hypnosis for entertainment purposes, for so many misconceptions can arise from what is seen to be some kind of controlling magic.

The first consideration has to be the subject and his/her susceptibility, and the second his/her state of mind and general state of health, including depressive tendencies, epilepsy and even psychotic tendencies etc., etc..

How on earth can a stage hypnotist have knowledge of these so important factors before he begins messing with their subconscious? It is imperative that he implement a considered means of carefully vetting his subjects.

Be warned: before hypnotising anyone, it is absolutely essential that the subject's personal history be investigated, for it is a fact that cases of damage levelled at stage hypnotists have invariably revealed that subject had problems before the event.

I myself have had the experience of having to help people whom I term "victims" of stage hypnosis, who have been traumatised by their experience. Without exception, they have proved to be people who had problems to begin with, and the experience of the stage show has served to heighten their insecurities and feelings of lack of control. They should never have got past a realistic vetting procedure.

Some clients express a real concern when beginning therapy regarding the all-important matter of control. Invariably, the source of their concern is their experience either as the "victim" or as a spectator at a stage show. It takes time to explain the reasoning behind the pronouncement that "Nobody can control the mind of another", and I would guess that many hours of my time have been wasted in this fruitless exercise. I would prefer that my time be utilised more effectively therapeutically.

Those who are selected by the stage hypnotist are the most susceptible that he can find, those who will perform to order. He does not want those who will provide a challenge to his "powers". Those he picks are, in the first instance volunteers, because they are not concerned with the fact that they will be made to look silly. They want to be the centre of attention, and are willing to subject themselves to the ridiculous suggestions which will be the content of the show.

If they were not willing to accept the suggestions of the hypnotist - perhaps because the suggestions fell outside their normal moral parameters, or were dangerous – they would simply be shocked out of trance if in fact hypnotised and refuse to comply. The embarrassment that can result from a suggestion that someone perform sometimes lewd and even disgusting acts is real. It may just be that the young woman who begins to remove her clothing in line with a suggestion by the hypnotist is in fact acting out one of her fantasies.

The question as to whether or not she is acting within her normal moral constraints then does become somewhat difficult. Inhibitions are certainly affected within the trance state.

What a mind-bending thought, that you or I could in fact control the mind of another. Surely every hypnotist in the land with just a modicum of skill and knowledge would become extremely rich in a very short time, as bank managers emptied their vaults at a simple suggestion! The proposal is simply too ridiculous and not worthy of the time and concern that, sadly, it commands.

I am not opposed to stage hypnotism to such a degree as those who would like to see it banned; there are some performers who are extremely careful and do ensure that they do not cause any harm, by means of vetting those who volunteer to come up on stage. I would personally like to see strict, enforceable guidelines laid down so that every person calling himself a hypnotist should be licensed within stringent requirements as to qualification. I have no doubt that the debate will continue.

As a therapist, you will find yourself in the privileged position of being trusted by people who sometimes feel that they have no reason at all to extend their trust to anyone. I would suggest that you owe it to the profession, to those who will be your clients, and then to yourself, to be the best that you can, keeping an open mind.

We cannot both judge others from within the constraints of our own experience and then allow them to be responsible for their own life. We are not advisors and how can we be, when the advice given usually begins with "If I were you ..."?

We are not that person, and we never can stand in their shoes, or experience in the way that they do, or feel their pain. The most valuable thing we can offer is the help that they require to help themselves better understand, and restore in them the faith that they need in their own abilities and capacities to make the judgements and decisions which are right for them; to help them gain that confidence which tells us all that it really is okay to be who we are.

Bibliography

Andreas, Steve & Andreas, Connirae:
   Change Your Mind And Keep The Change.
   Real People Press, 1987

Anson, Barrie:
   Holism Homeopathy Healing And The Hereafter.
   Wessex Aquarian, 1992

Bandler, Richard:
   Using Your Brain ... For A Change.
   Real People Press, 1985

Bandler, Richard & Grinder, John:
   Trance-formations: Neuro-Linguistic Programming and the Structure Of Hypnosis.
   Real People Press, 1981

Bandler, Richard & Grinder, John:
   Patterns Of The Hypnotic Techniques Of Milton H. Erickson M.D..
   Metamorphous Press, 1975

Charlesworth, Edward A. & Nathan, Ronald G.:
   Stress Management: A Comprehensive Guide To Wellness.
   Ballantine Books, 1985

Charlesworth, Edward A. & Nathan, Ronald G.:
   Stress Management: A Conceptual And Procedural Guide.
   Biobehavioral Books, 1980

Citrenbaum, Charles M., King, Mark E. & Cohen, William A.:
   Modern Clinical Hypnosis for Habit Control.
   W W Norton & Company, 1985

Dilts, Robert:
   Changing Belief Systems With NLP.
   Meta Publications, 1984

Dilts, Robert, Grinder, John, Bandler, Richard & DeLozier, Judith:
   Neuro-Linguistic Programming Volume I: The Study Of The Structure Of Submodalities.
   Meta Publications, 1980

Edgette, John H. & Edgette, Janet Sasson:
  The Handbook Of Hypnotic Phenomena In Psychotherapy/
  Brunner/Mazel Inc.,1995

Elman, Dave:
  Hypnotherapy.
  Westwood Publishing Company, 1964

Erickson, Milton H. & Rossi, Ernest L.:
  Hypnotherapy: An Exploratory Casebook.
  Irvington Publishers Inc.,1979

Gibson, H. B. & Heap, Michael :
  Hypnosis In Therapy.
  Lawrence Erlbaum Associates Inc., 1997

Hammond, D. Corydon (Editor):
  Handbook Of Hypnotic Suggestion And Metaphor.
  W W Norton & Company, 1990

Havens, Ronald A. (Editor):
  The Wisdom Of Milton H. Erickson: Volume I, Hypnosis & Hypnotherapy.
  Irvington Publishers Inc., 1996

Havens, Ronald A. (Editor):
  The Wisdom Of Milton H. Erickson: Volume II, Human Behavior & Psychotherapy.
  Irvington Publishers Inc., 1996

Havens, Ronald A. & Walters, Catherine:
  Hypnotherapy Scripts: A Neo-Erickson Approach To Persuasive Healing.
  Brunner/Mazel Inc., 1989

Hilgard, Ernest R. & Hilgard, Josephine R.:
  Hypnosis In The Relief Of Pain.
  Brunner/Mazel Inc.,1994

Kennedy, Eugene & Charles, Sarah:
  On Becoming A Counselor.
  Crossroad Publishing Company, 1977

Kopp, Richard R.:
  Metaphor Therapy: Using Client-Generated Metaphors In Psychotherapy.
  Brunner/Mazel Inc.,1995

Knight, Brian & Carr-Jones, Michael:
  Love, Sex & Hypnosis.
  Chessnut Press,1992

Lankton, Stephen R. & Lankton, Carol H.:
  The Answer Within: A Clinical Framework Of Ericksonian Therapy.
  Brunner/Mazel Inc., 1983

Mills, Joyce C. & Crowley, Richard J.:
  Therapeutic Metaphors For Children And The Child Within.
  Brunner/Mazel Inc.,1986

O'Hanlon, William Hudson:
  Taproots: Underlying Principles Of Milton Erickson's Therapy And Hypnosis.
  W W Norton & Company, 1987

Orbach, Susie:
  Fat is a Feminist Issue.
  Berkeley Publishing Group, 1987

Tebbetts, Charles:
  Self Hypnosis And Other Mind-Expanding Techniques.
  Westwwod Publishing Company Inc., 1987

Waxman, David:
  Hartland's Medical And Dental Hypnosis (Third Edition).
  Bailliere Tindall1995

Yapko, Michael:
  Trancework: An Introduction To The Practice Of Clinical Hypnosis.
  Brunner/Mazel Inc., 1990

Videotape Acknowledgements:

Hypnotism Training Film # 50 .... Gil Boyne 1991

Six Step Reframing .... Connirae Andreas 1992

The Swish Pattern .... Steve & Connirae Andreas 1986

Hypnotic Inductions .... Richard Bandler 1987

Another title from

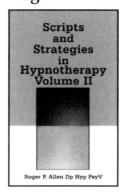

Crown House Publishing
www.crownhouse.co.uk

Scripts and Strategies in Hypnotherapy
Volume II
Roger P. Allen

More indispensable scripts for hypnotherapists. Covers inductions,
deepeners and actual scripts and strategies for a wide range of
problems. In particular, the book contains a very comprehensive
section on smoking cessation. Other areas covered are stress,
amnesia, anxiety, panic attacks, depression, low self-esteem,
nail-biting, weight loss, enuresis in children and dealing with
bereavement. Includes some of the most popular scripts from
Volume I.

"[There is a] wealth of new material to be found within the pages of
the current volume ... All in all, Roger Allen has contributed
another source of scripts and script ideas that sits comfortably with
the first volume and consequently should find a place on every
hypnotherapist's book shelf."
– *Peter Mabbutt DHyp (Dist), FBSCH*

HARDBACK   208 PAGES   ISBN: 1899836691

USA & Canada *orders to:*

Crown House Publishing
P.O. Box 2223, Williston, VT 05495-2223, USA
Tel: 877-925-1213, Fax: 802-864-7626
www.CHPUS.com

Australasia *orders to:*

Footprint Books Pty Ltd
101 McCarrs Creek Road, P.O. Box 418, Church Point
Sydney NSW 2105, Australia
Tel: +61 2 9997 3973, Fax: +61 2 9997 3185
E-mail: footprintbooks@ozmail.com.au

UK & Rest of World *orders to:*

The Anglo American Book Company Ltd.
Crown Buildings, Bancyfelin, Carmarthen, Wales SA33 5ND
Tel: +44 (0)1267 211880/211886, Fax: +44 (0)1267 211882
E-mail: books@anglo-american.co.uk
www.anglo-american.co.uk

100

BEST SELLING
ALBUMS OF THE

80s

100
BEST SELLING
ALBUMS OF THE
80s

Peter Dodd   Justin Cawthorne   Chris Barrett   Dan Auty

This 2009 edition published by 3C Publishing Ltd by arrangement with Amber Books Ltd.

3C Publishing Ltd
Sky House
Raans Road
Amersham
Bucks, HP6 6JQ

Editorial and design by:
Amber Books Ltd
Bradley's Close
74–77 White Lion St
London N1 9PF
United Kingdom
www.amberbooks.co.uk

ISBN: 978-1-906842-06-2

Project Editor: Tom Broder
Design: Colin Hawes
Picture Research: Natasha Jones
Consultant: Roger Watson

ACKNOWLEDGEMENTS

Thanks to the following for help with supplying the albums as well as for their invaluable industry knowledge:
Reckless Records (www.reckless.co.uk), Soho, London
Flashback (www.flashback.co.uk), Islington, London
Golden Grooves (www.goldengroovesrecords.com), Old Street, London
Haggle (www.hagglevinyl.com), Islington, London
The Music and Video Exchange, Notting Hill, London
Stage and Screen, Notting Hill, London
Beanos (www.beanos.co.uk)

Copyrights held by:
Virgin Music: The Rolling Stones, page 19

Printed in China

Contents

Editor's foreword

The ranking of the 100 best-selling albums of the 1980s listed in the following pages is based upon the number of platinum and multi-platinum sales awards that each album has achieved, as certified by the Recording Industry Association of America (RIAA) and the British Phonographic Industry (BPI). The RIAA platinum award represents sales of at least 1,000,000 albums, while the BPI platinum certification is awarded for sales of at least 300,000 albums.

In an industry not always noted for the accuracy of its published sales figures, these awards are one of the most effective and reliable measures of sales success, providing a consistent way to rate the relative position of the decade's best-selling albums. These figures also have the advantage – unlike similar lists based on chart position – of showing aggregate album sales from the date of first release right up until the present day.

Ranking of equal sellers

Where two or more albums have the same sales total they are arranged by date of release, with the most recent album released ranked highest, since its sales are stronger relative to time spent

on the market. Bruce Springsteens's 1980 album *The River*, for example, has had almost a decade longer to achieve its sales of 5,100,000 than Don Henley's 1989 release *The End Of Innocence*, and is therefore ranked lower in the list.

Compilations and soundtracks

Compilation or greatest hits albums are not included in this list, which is why the Bob Marley compilation album, *Legend*, which has won a staggering 10 RIAA platinum awards since it's posthumous 1984 release, does not feature. However live albums and original movie or musical soundtracks, where all of the songs have been collected together or recorded specifically for the album, are included. The soundtrack to the 1983 film *The Big Chill*, for example, introduced a new generation to Motown classics such as Marvin Gaye's 'Heard It Through The Grapevine' and Aretha Franklin's '(You Me Feel) Like A Natural Woman'.

US and international album sales

The lists in this book are based on both US and UK album sales; the BPI award scheme was only introduced in the mid-1970s, making this the first decade where it is possible to use the awards to calculate UK album sales. The sheer size of the North-American album market relative to that of other regions means that the list is inevitably weighted toward US top sellers. Nonetheless, UK artists are well represented, with both Phil Collins and Dire Straits making it into the Top Ten.

Facts and figures

The appendices provide a breakdown of some of the most interesting facts and figures found throughout this book. You can find out which artists have the most albums in the list and who are the highest-ranking US and UK acts. You can see which albums have won the most Grammy awards or contain the most Number One singles, what were the best-selling soundtracks and live albums, and which record labels were the most successful of the decade.

Alongside tributes to old favourites there are enough surprises to keep the most dedicated music buff guessing and stimulate plenty of lively discussion. Country-rockers Alabama's 1982 release *Mountain Music*, for example, comfortably outsold Prince's decade-defining album *1999*, which was released later the same year. The albums are illustrated using a mixture of the US and UK sleeve designs – a selection that includes some of the most iconic images of the decade.

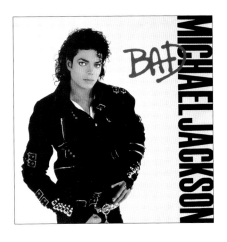

Michael Jackson's 1987 album *Bad* contains five tracks that went on to become Number One singles, more than any other record among the 100 best-selling albums. However it is *Bad*'s predecessor, *Thriller*, that has won the most Grammy awards.

The Best-Selling Albums of the 1980s

At the beginning of the 1980s, it looked as if the mainstream album market might still be savaged by punk rock. But with the new decade, came the realization that the punk revolution was too insular ever to maintain strong album sales.

Prime punk purveyors, the Sex Pistols, played selected American venues in a flurry of publicity, but interest soon waned. Punk was just too plain nasty for America. Sure, the US had pioneered rock 'n' roll anarchy, but Elvis never cursed in public and Bill Haley looked like a smartly dressed businessman. The US had the Ramones and other punk bands, but they never really identified with Britain's punk ethos, nurtured by the economic conditions and social divisions present in the UK at that time.

Pop grows up

Because of the huge impact made by British bands such as The Beatles in the 1960s, the US never quite gave up its image of Britain as a magical mystery tour, where London was always swinging. The anarchic Sex Pistols were too extreme to sustain anything more than fleeting curiosity value, but album sales in the 1980s showed America's renewed faith in British pop music. Spearheaded by Culture Club, Spandau Ballet and Duran Duran, the Brit-inspired 'new romantic' movement helped re-establish quality music ideals and provided the perfect accompaniment to new hopeful times.

But album sales during this decade also reflected a taste for more established and mature sounds. In the 1980s, pop music's paranoid obsession with youth greatly disappeared. The generation born in the post-war years demanded music to satisfy and reflect its ever-maturing aspirations, traumas and fears.

In 1981, Phil Collins' album *Face Value* tapped into this market, entering the UK album chart at Number One and spending 274 weeks there. Most of the songs on *Face Value* were inspired by the break-up of Collins' marriage, and the album became essential listening for angst-ridden divorcees. Collins re-wrote 'How Can You Sit There', a song from the *Face Value* sessions, as the theme for the movie *Against All Odds*. It became his first million-selling single, and earned him an Oscar nomination. Collins was the first of two drummers to enjoy massive solo success in the 1980s: Don Henley of the Eagles also charted strongly with *The End of the Innocence*.

They might be giants

The 1980s was a profitable era for many bands who had come to prominence in the previous decade. Even though it had been predicted that the anarchic days of the late 1970s would sweep away established acts, album sales for music's old guard continued to be healthy.

At the start of the 1980s, Pink Floyd's album *The Wall* dominated the charts. Released at the very end of 1979 it went on to top the US album chart for 15 weeks, ushering in the new decade. A 1982 movie version of *The Wall* was also made, directed by Alan Parker and starring Bob Geldof, organizer of 1985's *Live Aid.* This star-studded concert, staged in London and Philidephia, raised millions of dollars to fight famine in Ethiopia and became a defining cultural moment of the 1980s.

West-Coast AOR champions, Fleetwood Mac, continued to do well with *Tango in the Night*, and the Rolling Stones were well up the album chart with 1981's *Tattoo You*. Billy Joel built on his previous successes with *An Innocent Man*, while veteran soul crooner Lionel Richie could comfortably bathe in the afterglow of his massive 1983 hit *Can't Slow Down*. Another band forged in the fiery crucible of the late 1970s, The Police, continued to be a major force, especially with their 1983 album *Synchronicity*, based on psychologist Carl Jung's theories of coincidence.

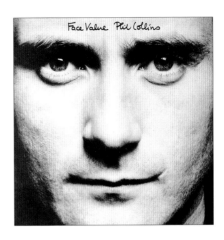

Former Genesis drummer Phil Collins' 1981 solo album *Face Value* appealed to the hopes and aspirations of the baby-boomer generation coming to terms with approaching middle age.

Video killed the radio star

During the 1980s, albums evolved beyond simple pieces of vinyl sold in a nice cover. Video meant that albums became multi-media packages; images and songs shaped and defined as much by film as they once had been by music alone. The video age truly began with the launch of the MTV network in 1981. Many up-and-coming bands were quick to realise the potential of MTV – exposure on the network could substantially fuel single and album sales. By 1983, no major record label was complete without its own video department.

Michael Jackson was one artist who was quick to appreciate the power of video, which became not only an entertainment medium, but a vehicle for social change. The video for 'Billie Jean' was, surprisingly, the first video by an African-American artist to receive major air time on MTV. It paved the way for other black artists to gain the recognition they deserved.

The 1980s were Jackson's golden years, a time when he redefined dance music and re-energized it. Nothing Jackson has done since has quite surpassed the dance-floor filling, pumping passion of *Thriller*. Released in December 1982, *Thriller* was Number One in almost every western country, including the US, where it spent 37 weeks at the top of the album

chart. The album sold over 1,000,000 copies in Los Angeles alone and spawned seven US Top-Ten singles. Nominated for a staggering 12 Grammy awards, *Thriller* has gone on to become the most successful chart album of all time.

Jackson's video for the 'Thriller' single was a camp horror classic, complete with a chilling voice-over from horror-film veteran Vincent Price. After the 'Thriller' video was aired on MTV, more than 400,000 copies of the album were sold in less than seven days.

Movie magic

Just as 1980s pop music came to feed off the visual thrills of MTV, many of the top-selling albums of the decade were film soundtracks. In *Top Gun*, Tom Cruise seduced Kelly McGillis over a thunderous soundtrack that featured the Righteous Brothers and Berlin. The glossy, adrenaline-fuelled movie acted as an extended promotional video for the album, which went on to sell over 9,000,000 copies in the US alone.

The title track for *Footloose*, the tale of a musically repressed town in the mid-west coming alive to rock 'n' roll, was written by veteran musician Kenny Loggins. Among the other songs was Foreigner's 'Waiting For A Girl Like You'. *Flashdance*, the story of a female steelworker who becomes a nightclub dancer, made over $97,000,000 when released in 1983. Television also proved a fertile medium for pop music. The popular *Miami Vice* TV series was like one long MTV video, and the soundtrack album produced lucrative sales. Other successful albums included U2's soundtrack to their documentary film, *Rattle And Hum*, and Prince's soundtrack to his masterpiece *Purple Rain*.

Goodbye to vinyl

Another startling new innovation was the compact disc. Introduced in 1982, CDs promised listeners clearer, distortion-free, sound. Although CDs would not dominate the album market until the 1990s, by 1989 around 28 percent of households in the US had a CD player and around 288,000,000 compact discs were sold each year.

But the CD wasn't the greatest rival to the LP during the 1980s – for much of the decade it was the tape cassette that threatened to kill off vinyl completely. The cassette offered music buyers unrivalled convenience – the introduction of the Sony Walkman in 1979 meant people could listen to their favourite music on the move – and could record music as well as play it. These advantages made tapes the format of choice for many listeners during the 1980s and by 1983 cassette albums outsold vinyl LPs in the record shops (although CD sales would in turn surpass

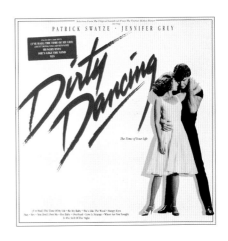

With the release of *Dirty Dancing* in 1987, millions of teenage girls dreamed of being swept off their feet by Patrick Swayze. The accompanying album – especially the hit single '(I've Had) The Time Of My Life' – provided the perfect soundtrack for their fantasies.

sales of tape by the early 1990s). This new technology offered many advantages over the humble LP, but there were many record buyers who regretted the passing of the vinyl record's heyday and missed the pleasure and anticipation of opening a gatefold 12-inch album sleeve and hearing the scratching, crackling noises of a needle lowered on to vinyl.

Back to basics

The 1980s may have been an era for revolutionary new media technology, but many albums continued to reflect traditional rock 'n' roll ethics. Of all modern American guitar heroes, none filled the role of working-class kid made good better than Bruce Springsteen. Released in June 1984, *Born in the U.S.A.* was both a celebration and an uncompromising examination of American life. The album spent seven weeks at the top of the US chart.

The 1980s saw a triumvirate of classic rock albums released by new bands. Def Leppard, a group of young hopefuls from Sheffield, UK, were once so broke that they all shared the same bed in dingy motels when they were gigging. By 1987, following a series of grinding tours, Def Leppard had become stadium-rock kings. Three years in the making, *Hysteria* hit the US album chart at Number Ten in March 1988.

Meanwhile, a former shoe salesman, Jon Bon Jovi, had been moulding his band into stadium headliners. The 1980s were the classic years for stadium rock, with large tours, masses of equipment and capacity crowds. It may have been the video age, but there was nothing to surpass a live concert on a hot summer's evening. Bon Jovi's album *Slippery When Wet* was an anthem-filled pop-metal masterpiece. Released in 1986, by the end of the following year it had sold 8,000,000 copies in the US.

There was no stopping AC/DC either. After the demise of singer Bon Scott, who died tragically in 1980, the band recruited former Geordie frontman Brian Johnson, and came storming onto the album chart with *Back In Black*.

Wild boys

Guns N' Roses were the real bad boys of rock in the 1980s. Although their career was unruly and controversial, the band produced plenty of magnificent work, including their 1987 release *Appetite For Destruction*. In 1989, Guns N' Roses became the first band for more than 10 years to have two albums simultaneously in the US album Top Five. The 1980s also saw Ozzy Osbourne begin a new phase in his long-lived and dexterous career when he left Black Sabbath and formed Blizzard of Ozz. The band's 1980 debut album, *Blizzard Of Ozz*, and the follow up, *Diary Of A Madman*, both went platinum.

Starlets and divas

Like Hollywood, the album charts of the 1980s were full of fresh-faced starlets desperate to fulfil their dreams. Madonna arrived in New York with a few dollars in her pocket but a wealth of talent. A true child of the video age, Madonna knew perfectly how to manipulate the medium. By the end of the decade, with hit albums such as *Like A Virgin* and *True Blue* under her belt, Madonna had become a music, film and fashion icon. Because of her massive exposure, no girl's wardrobe was complete without a selection of micro skirts and flashy jewellery.

The 1980s was the era when two other pop divas, Whitney Houston and Janet Jackson, also established themselves. In 1985, Whitney's eponymous album spent more than 100 weeks on the UK album chart and it topped the US charts in March 1986. In October 1989, Janet Jackson's album *Rhythm Nation 1814* – inspired by the year in which Francis Scott Key wrote the Star Spangled Banner – began a four-week stint at the Number One position.

The 1980s also saw something of a rebirth for Tina Turner. Her career lull had cost her dearly: owing more than $300,000, she had been

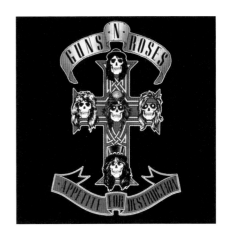

Guns N' Roses stormed the 1980s album charts with characteristic thunder and attitude. Their 15,000,000-selling debut *Appetite For Destruction* helped breathe new life into hard rock and metal.

reduced to performing cheap cabaret gigs just to survive. Then she met up with Australian promoter Roger Davies and turned her life around. Released in summer 1984, Turner's comeback album, *Private Dancer*, stayed on the US album chart for almost a year.

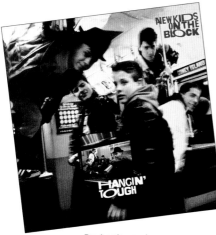

Boy bands were by no means a new phenomena in the 1980s, but New Kids On The Block provided the genre with new impetus and paved the way for groups like the Backstreet Boys in the 1990s.

Going up and moving down

The 1980s album charts witnessed the birth of many long-term success stories, one of the most enduring being stadium-filling country superstar Garth Brooks. His 1989 release, simply titled *Garth Brooks*, began a run of multi-platinum albums that would turn him into one of the most successful artists in any genre by the 1990s.

The decade also saw a number of artists who would fail to make much impact in the future. Pop balladeer Tracy Chapman failed to capitalize on the strength of her debut, while Paula Abdul faired little better after the success of *Forever Your Girl*. Tiffany almost sank without trace after the release of her first album, as did Milli Vanilli when it was discovered that their songs – and their singing – were not all their own. Australian band Men at Work, who had scored a massive hit single with 'Down Under', quickly faded after the release of their second album, *Cargo*.

The new boys

Music purists sneered that New Kids On The Block, the first of what seemed to be a never-ending stream of boy bands, were cynically manufactured. Other commentators questioned whether any successful pop band hadn't owed at least something to clever management and subtle media manipulation.

But not all boy bands were so squeaky clean. The Beastie Boys were three middle-class white rappers who had the guts to steal pieces of black music culture, using sampled cuts from artists such as James Brown to start a rap music revolution. Mega album-selling band Aerosmith were also exploring these intriguing new sounds. In one of the most unlikely combinations of the decade they teamed up with Run DMC for 'Walk This Way', a fusion of rap and heavy metal that became a spectacular success.

Music in the material world

The 1980s was a vigorous time for album sales. The record industry had lived through the trauma of the late 1970s and realised that it could survive. The threat posed by independent labels had largely disappeared and there was plenty of new talent to draw on, much of which would survive well into the next decade and beyond. Album sales in the 1980s were so healthy that the Recording Industry Association of America (RIAA) decided to institute a new honour for artists whose album sales were particularly strong, introducing multi-platinum status for those selling 2,000,000 units or more. The advent of video and CDs made the 1980s a challenging era for pop music – but the record industry took full advantage of living in a material world.

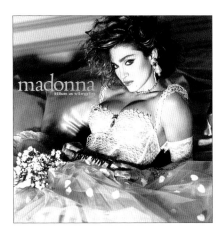

Madonna enjoyed a string of hit singles and albums through the 1980s. Tracks like 'Material Girl', from her 1984 album *Like A Virgin*, perfectly summed up the go-getting mood of the decade.

100 Blizzard Of Ozz

| • Album sales: 4,100,000 | • Release date: December 1980 |

The first project after his acrimonious 1978 departure from Black Sabbath turned out to be the biggest-selling album of Ozzy Osbourne's long career. Much of his initial solo success can be attributed to guitarist Randy Rhodes. Formerly of Quiet Riot, Rhodes formed the nexus of Osbourne's new band, also called Blizzard Of Ozz, featuring Bob Daisley on bass and Lee Kerslake (ex-Uriah Heep) on drums. Credit should also be given to Sharon Arden, Osbourne's future wife, who had begun managing him and guiding his career.

The presence of the track 'Mr Crowley', said to be inspired by the Satanist Aleister Crowley, guaranteed the controversy factor was in place. It was destined to became one of his most popular solo songs, along with 'Crazy Train', 'Suicide Solution' and 'Revelation (Mother Earth)'.

Osbourne supported Blizzard Of Ozz with a concert tour in which he performed new solo material as well as standards from his days with Black Sabbath. Although 'Crazy Train' and 'Mr Crowley' were released as singles, neither was commercially successful. Blizzard Of Ozz is one of very few amongst the 100 best-selling albums of the 1980s to have acheived such great sales without the benefit of a Top 40 single.

Number One singles:
None

Grammy awards:
None

Label: US: Jet-CBS;
UK: CBS

Recorded in:
Surrey, UK

Personnel:
Ozzy Osbourne
Randy Rhoads

Don Airey
Bob Daisley
Lee Kerslake
Mark Lennon
John Shanks
Danny Saber
Robert Trujillo
Mike Bordin

Producers:
Ozzy Osbourne
Randy Rhoads
Bob Daisley
Lee Kerslake

1. I Don't Know (5:14)
2. Crazy Train (4:50)
3. Goodbye to Romance (5:36)
4. Dee (0:50)
5. Suicide Solution (4:16)
6. Mr. Crowley (4:56)
7. No Bone Movies (3:58)
8. Revelation (Mother Earth) (6:09)
9. Steal Away (The Night) (3:30)

Total album length: 39 minutes

Ozzy Osbourne

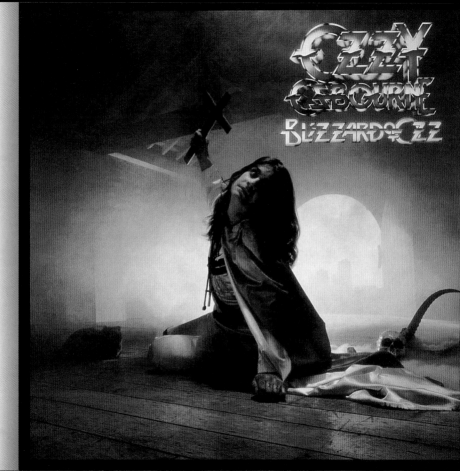

Tattoo You

| **Album sales:** 4,100,000 | **Release date:** August 1981 |

In a career as long and as illustrious as the one enjoyed by the Rolling Stones, it would be forgivable to dismiss *Tattoo You* as simply yet another Stones album. Not so, as sales indicate. Like its predecessor, 1980s *Emotional Rescue*, it's something of a housekeeping exercise involving the rerecording of many unreleased songs, some of which stretched back to 1972. The resulting *Tattoo You* topped the chart in the US (giving the band their last Number One album in that country) and reached Number Two in the UK.

Split into fast and slow sides, the album kicks off with 'Start Me Up', the first single. Reaching Number Two in the US (Number 7 in the UK), it provided the Stones with their biggest hit since 'Miss You' in 1978. The softer 'Waiting On A Friend', featuring Sonny Rollins on sax, acheived Number 13 (Number 50 in the UK), was helped by a popular B-side, 'Little T & A', with Keith Richards on vocals. 'Hang Fire' reached Number 20 in the US, but failed to chart in the UK.

The Stones embarked on a world-wide tour in support of *Tattoo You*, captured in the 1982 live *Still Life* album. The popularity of *Tattoo You*, combined with the highly successful tour, prompted the release of the compilation album *Sucking In The Seventies* in late 1981.

Number One singles:
None

Grammy awards:
None

Label: US & UK:
Rolling Stones

Recorded in:
Various locations

Personnel:
Mick Jagger
Keith Richards
Ron Wood
Bill Wyman
Charlie Watts
Mick Taylor
Sonny Rollins
Wayne Perkins

Producers:
Mick Jagger
Keith Richards

1 Start Me Up (3:31)
2 Hang Fire (2:30)
3 Slave (6:34)
4 Little T & A (3:23)
5 Black Limousine (3:31)
6 Neighbours (3:30)
7 Worried About You (5:16)
8 Tops (3:45)
9 Heaven (4:21)
10 No Use In Crying (3:24)
11 Waiting On A Friend (4:34)

Total album length: 44 minutes

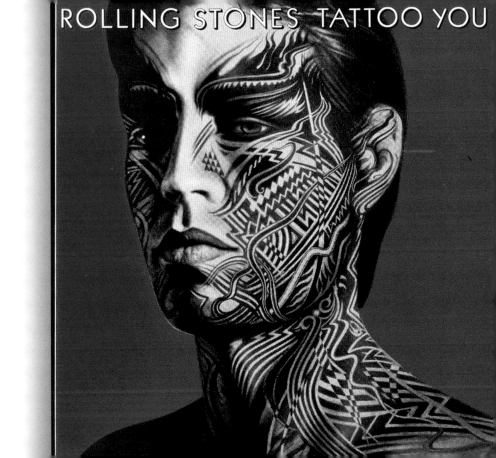

98 For Those About To Rock We Salute You

| • **Album sales:** 4,100,000 | • **Release date:** November 1981 |

It's quite an achievement for a major rock band to have a fatality in the front man department and bounce back bigger than ever – but that's exactly what happened with AC/DC. In 1980 vocalist Bon Scott died, according to the coroner, by drinking himself to death. Undaunted, the band recruited a replacement in the form of Brian Johnson, and returned to the fray with 'Back In Black' which would prove to be their greatest success. 'For Those About to Rock We Salute You' simply continued the tradition although it would also prove in time to be the climax of their commercial clout with less successful material following.

By now Johnson was on his second album and had fully found his feet as the AC/DC

frontman delivering powerhouse vocals on the hits 'Let's Get It Up' and the title track.

Befitting the album title, the sleeve featured a cannon and cannon fire was soon a staple of the live show with 'For Those About to Rock (We Salute You)' becoming classic live fodder.

Ultimately, perhaps, the sad departure of Bon Scott was more profoundly affecting than first thought. Whatever the reason, after *For Those About To Rock We Salute You*, AC/DC started to experience diminishing commercial returns.

Number One singles:
None

Grammy awards: None

Label: US & UK: Atlantic

Recorded in:
Paris, France

Personnel:
Brian Johnson
Angus Young
Malcolm Young
Cliff Williams
Phil Rudd

Producers:
Robert John 'Mutt' Lange

1 For Those About To Rock (We Salute You) (5:43)
2 I Put The Finger On You (3:25)
3 Let's Get It Up (3:53)
4 Inject The Venom (3:30)
5 Snowballed (3:23)
6 Evil Walks (4:23)
7 C.O.D. (3:19)
8 Breaking The Rules (4:23)
9 Night Of The Long Knives (3:25)
10 Spellbound (4:30)

Total album length: 40 minutes

AC/DC

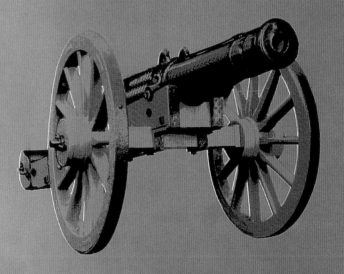

AC⚡DC

FOR THOSE ABOUT TO ROCK

97 Asia

| • Album sales: 4,100,000 | • Release date: March 1982 |

A 1970s-style supergroup made up of refugees from Yes, King Crimson, Emerson Lake & Palmer and Buggles hardly had the makings of a top-selling act in the post-punk early 1980s. However, Asia silenced their critics when their eponymous debut album spent two months atop the charts. What separated Asia from their indulgent forbears was that they had a pop sensibility largely courtesy of keyboardist and former Buggle Geoff Downes, who brought with him some of the quirkiness of his former band's 1979 single 'Video Killed The Radio Star'.

The Top Five US hit single 'Heat Of The Moment' sealed the success of *Asia*, taking it beyond the arena of old school progressive rock fans and into the mainstream. 'Only Time Will Tell' provided a second US Top 20 hit, and other album tracks became familiar radio plays. Shortly after its release, *Asia* reached Number One on the US charts, a position it held for nine straight weeks. The new supergroup received a much more muted reception on the other side of the Atlantic, where 'Heat Of The Moment' and 'Only Time Will Tell' peaked at Number 46 and Number 54 respectively.

While Asia may not have been the hippest act of the moment, in the US some clearly found their slightly anachronistic yet eminently worthwhile efforts a desirable alternative to the dominant trends of the time.

Number One singles: None	**Personnel:** Steve Howe
	John Wetton
Grammy awards: None	Geoffrey Downes
	Carl Palmer
Label: US & UK: Geffen	
	Producers:
Recorded in: N/A	Mike 'Clay' Stone

1 Heat Of The Moment (3:54)
2 Only Time Will Tell (4:48)
3 Sole Survivor (4:52)
4 One Step Closer (4:18)
5 Time Again (4:47)
6 Wildest Dreams (5:11)
7 Without You (5:07)
8 Cutting It Fine (5:40)
9 Here Comes The Feeling (5:43)

Total album length: 43 minutes

Asia

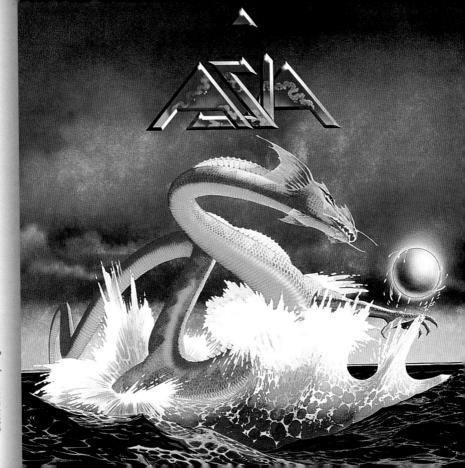

96 1999

• Album sales: 4,100,000 | **• Release date:** November 1982

Prince's next album, the soundtrack to the film *Purple Rain*, would blast him into rock megastardom, but in the meantime *1999* was a delicious appetiser for what was to come.

The precocious star who had insisted on total artistic control since he first signed to Warner, had already established that he was a major force to be reckoned with showing his considerable talents as a writer and musician coupled with a penchant for notoriety.

Now Prince had stepped up a gear and had moved into the realm of world-beating songwriting. An ambitious set, *1999* was the first of what would become many double-albums from Prince. It would also be the first to propel the artist into the Top Ten of the US singles chart. The first single, '1999', failed to do the trick, peaking at Number 44 in November 1982, but the second, 'Little Red Corvette', reached Number Six the following spring. Other singles followed, including 'Delirious', another Top Ten hit. Such was Prince's newfound popularity that a reissue of the title track made it to Number 12 in the summer of 1983.

The album went on to become Prince's best-selling to date, peaking at Number Nine on the US chart during an astonishing 125-week run.

Number One singles:
None

Grammy awards:
None

Label: US & UK: Warner

Recorded in:
Los Angeles, USA

Producer:
Prince

Personnel:
Prince
Brownmark
Lisa Coleman
Wendy Melvoin
Poochie
Vanity
The Count
Dez Dickerson
Jill Jones
Peggy McCreary
Jamie Starr

1   1999 (6:15)
2   Little Red Corvette (5:03)
3   Delirious (4:00)
4   Let's Pretend We're Married (7:21)
5   D.M.S.R. (8:17)
6   Automatic (9:28)
7   Something In The Water (Does Not Compute) (4:02)
8   Free (5:08)
9   Lady Cab Driver (8:19)
10 All The Critics Love U In New York (5:59)
11 International Lover (6:37)

Total album length: 70 minutes

Prince

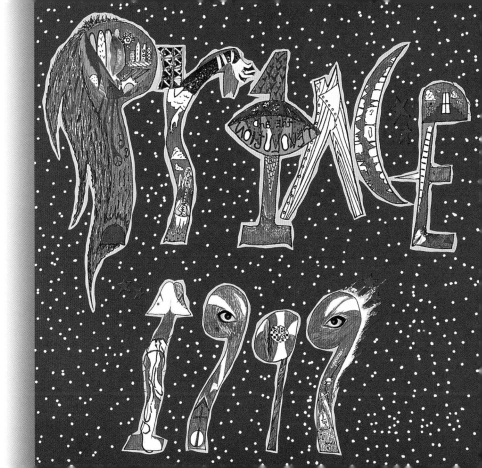

95 Miami Vice

| • **Album sales:** 4,100,000 | • **Release date:** June 1985 |

Czechoslovakian-born jazz-fusion keyboard player Jan Hammer was the man who provided the musical complement to the high-gloss slickness of the smash hit TV cop series *Miami Vice*. Probably one of the reasons the soundtrack fared so well is that the plotlines famously featured musical vignettes – almost music videos – as police officers Crockett (Don Johnson) and Tubbs (Philip Michael Thomas) went about their crime-bustin' business.

Hammer's original theme to the show earned a Number One single, a fairly rare event for an instrumental. All the other pieces were featured different episodes. Eagles founder Glenn Frey contributed two cuts, 'You Belong To The City' and 'Smuggler's Blues'. The latter, from his 1984 *Allnighter* album, inspired one of the episodes. Frey himself made a guest appearance in the show, a move which would lead to further acting roles for the singer, including appearances in the *Wiseguy* TV series.

Sales of the album were supported by the inclusion of two previous US hit singles, Phil Collins' 'In The Air Tonight' and Tina Turner offers 'Better Be Good To Me'.

Number One singles:
US: Miami Vice Theme

Grammy awards: Best pop instrumental performance (orchestra, group or soloist); Best instrumental composition

Label: US & UK: MCA

Recorded in:
Various locations

Personnel:
Jan Hammer
Glenn Frey
Chaka Khan
Phil Collins
Tina Turner
Grandmaster Melle Mel
Various other personnel

Producers:
Phil Collins
Jan Hammer
Joe Mardin
Leland Robinson

1 The Original Miami Vice Theme (Jan Hammer) (1:02)
2 Smuggler's Blues (Glenn Frey) (3:50)
3 Own The Night (Chaka Khan) (4:52)
4 You Belong To The City (Glenn Frey) (5:51)
5 In The Air Tonight (Phil Collins) (5:29)
6 Miami Vice (Jan Hammer) (2:28)
7 Vice (Grandmaster Melle Mel) (5:02)
8 Better Be Good To Me (Tina Turner) (5:11)
9 Flashback (Jan Hammer) (3:20)
10 Chase (Jan Hammer) (2:39)
11 Evan (Jan Hammer) (3:08)

Total album length: 43 minutes

Original TV Soundtrack

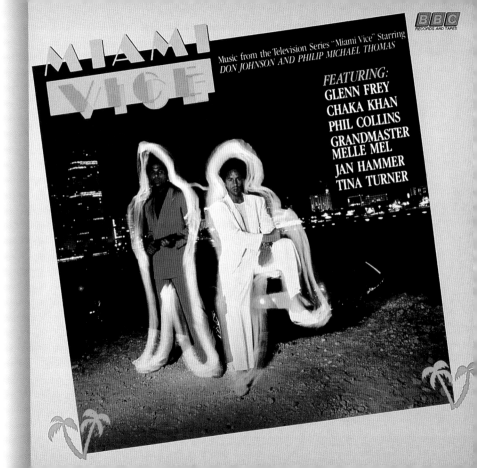

94 5150

| • Album sales: 4,100,000 | • Release date: March 1986 |

The single most significant factor about *5150*, Van Halen's first album since their hugely successful *1984*, is that it came one year after the departure of lead singer David Lee Roth. At first, the band considered using a different guest vocalist for each track, before settling on the goal of finding a permanent replacement for Roth. They settled on former Montrose vocalist Sammy Hagar, who had seen little commercial success in his long solo career.

Named after Eddie Van Halen's home studio, *5150* was a commercial success, providing the band with their first US Number One album (Number 16 in the UK). It remained on the *Billboard* album chart for a total of 64 weeks.

The album's first single, 'Why Can't This Be Love', gave Van Halen their second US Top Ten hit, while 'Dreams' and 'Love Walks In' both reached Number 22.

While Van Halen's fanbase was in turmoil about the change in vocalist and the new synthesizer driven sound, the more than healthy sales and a sell-out tour gave clear indication that Eddie Van Halen, guitar virtuoso and son of a Dutch bandleader, was still very much on track.

Number One singles:
None

Grammy awards:
None

Label: US & UK: Warner

Recorded in:
California, USA

Personnel:
Sammy Hagar
Eddie Van Halen
Michael Anthony
Alex Van Halen

Producers:
Mick Jones
Donn Landee
Sammy Hagar
Eddie Van Halen
Michael Anthony
Alex Van Halen

1 Good Enough (4:00)
2 Why Can't This Be Love? (3:45)
3 Get Up (4:35)
4 Dreams (4:54)
5 Summer Nights (5:04)
6 Best Of Both Worlds (4:49)
7 Love Walks In (5:09)
8 5150 (5:44)
9 Inside (5:02)

Total album length: 43 minutes

Van Halen

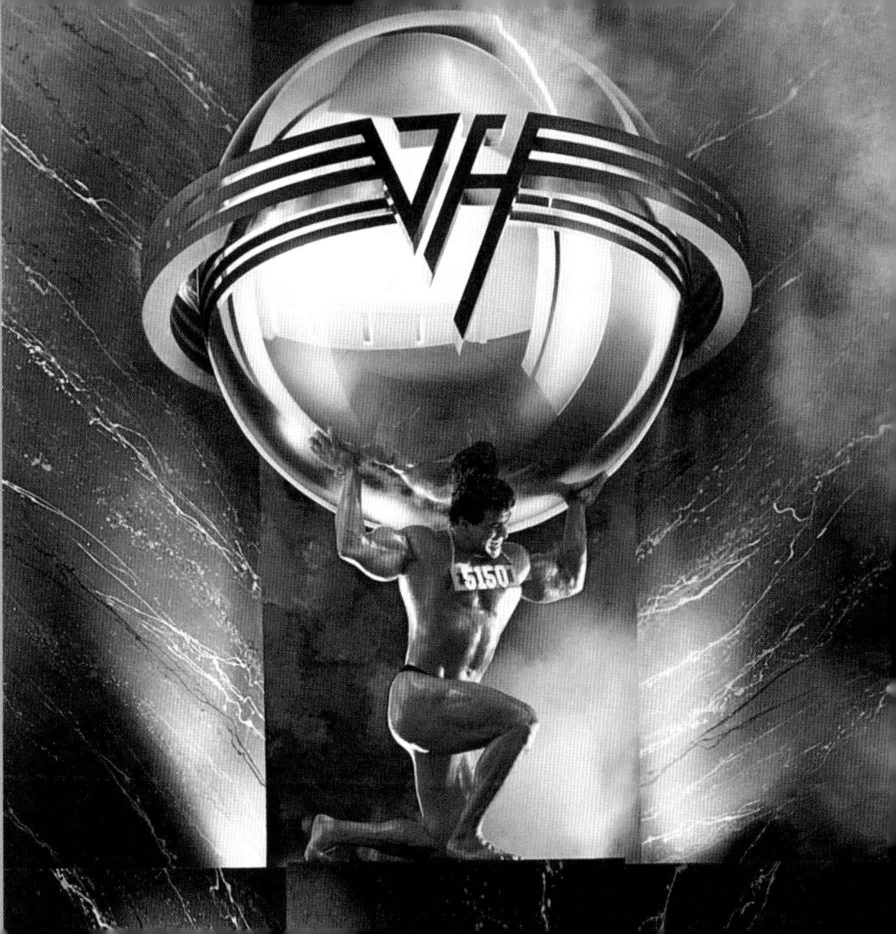

Sleeve artwork by Jeri McManus and Aaron Rapoport

93 Third Stage

| • Album sales: 4,100,000 | • Release date: September 1986 |

Not only is *Third Stage* a comment on the stages visited through life, where this album is concerned it was also a reference to the record itself, which arrived an extraordinary eight years after its predecessor, Boston's second album, *Don't Look Back*. By this time, only the original nucleus of vocalist Brad Delp and songwriter Tom Scholz remained. This served to prove that the duo owned the Boston sound as comparisons with their earlier sound abound.

Although arguably not as universally popular as their earlier work, *Third Stage* nevertheless saw sales nearly equal to *Don't Look Back*. Two months after its release, *Third Stage* reached Number One spot on the US album chart, a position it held for four weeks. That same month,

it brought the band its only chart-topping US single with 'Amanda'. The follow-up, 'We're Ready', was a Top Ten hit, while 'Can'tcha Say (You Believe in Me)' peaked at Number 20. received considerable less attention. A fourth single, 'Hollyann' failed to chart; Boston would never have another Top 40 single.

Clearly Scholz's quest for perfection is a significant feature in the Boston landscape. Fans of *Third Stage* would have to wait until 1994 before the band's next album, *Walk On*, was released. Sales of that album amounted to one million copies – a considerable number, but one that pales in comparison to the 17 million units sold of the band's debut album.

Number One singles:
US: Amanda

Grammy awards:
None

Label: US & UK: MCA

Recorded in:
Massachusetts, USA

Personnel:
Brad Delp
Tom Scholz
Jim Masdea
Gary Pihl

Producer:
Tom Scholz

1 Amanda (4:16)
2 We're Ready (3:53)
3 The Launch (3:00)
4 Cool The Engines (4:23)
5 My Destination (2:13)
6 A New World (0:36)
7 To Be A Man (3:33)
8 I Think I Like It (4:10)
9 Can'tcha Say (You Believe in Me): Still in (5:18)
10 Hollyann (5:18)

Total album length: 36:40

Boston

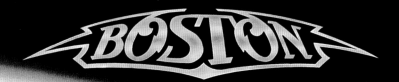

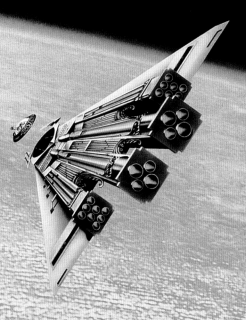

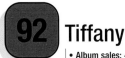

92 Tiffany

• **Album sales:** 4,100,000 • **Release date:** May 1987

Born in 1971, Tiffany became the youngest female artist to top the *Billboard* charts with a debut album. In her yet younger days Tiffany Renee Darwish, as she was then known, was pursuing a career as a country singer and was discovered by veteran Hoyt Axton while performing at a Los Angeles nightclub.

Later, under the guidance – or as some would say vice-like grip – of manager George Tobin, she secured a recording deal with MCA and turned her attention from country to bubblegum.

Following the release of *Tiffany*, she embarked on a concert tour of US shopping malls. Initially, the change of musical direction and unusual promotion produced no immediate results; 'Danny', the album's first single, failed to chart. However, by the autumn of 1987, 'I Think We're Alone Now', a cover of the Tommy James and the Shondells hit, was a US Number One single. Tiffany's career now snowballed pushing the album to the top of the charts, where it had the distinction of replacing Michael Jackson's *Bad*.

A follow-up single 'Could've Been' fared just as well as its predecessor, and her interpretation of the Lennon/McCartney standard 'I Saw Her Standing There' (as 'I Saw *Him* Standing There') provided a final hit from the album.

Number One singles: US & UK: I Think We're Alone Now; US: Could've Been

Grammy awards: None

Label: US & UK: MCA

Recorded in: N/A

Personnel:
Tiffany
Irving Azoff
Craig T Cooper
John Duarte
Richard Elliott
Steve Holroyd
Dann Huff
John Kerns
David Means
Steve Rucker
George Tobin
Carl Verheyen
Chuck Yamek
Bryan Rutter
Bill Smith
Ned McElroy
Valerie Trotter

Producer:
George Tobin

1 Should've Been Me (3:39)
2 Danny (4:00)
3 Spanish Eyes (3:56)
4 Feelings Of Forever (3:52)
5 Kid On A Corner (4:02)
6 I Saw Him Standing There (4:12)
7 Johnny's Got The Inside Moves (3:20)
8 Promises Made (4:50)
9 I Think We're Alone Now (3:47)
10 Could've Been (3:30)

Total album length: 39 minutes

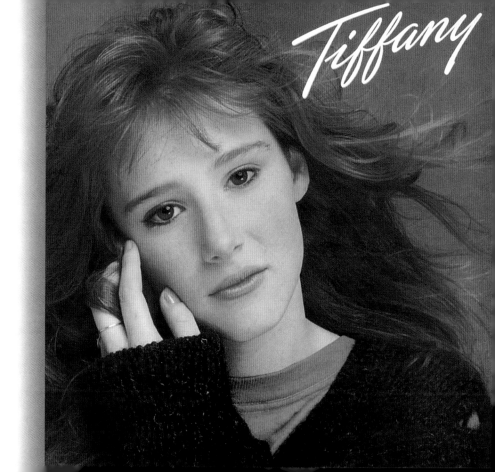

91 Open Up And Say... Ahh

| • **Album sales:** 4,100,000 | • **Release date:** May 1988 |

With the release of their debut album, *Look What The Cat Dragged In*, Harrisburg, Pennsylvannia's Poison found themselves rubbing shoulders with the likes of Bon Jovi and Def Leppard. The triple-platinum album produced three hit singles catapulted them to their lofty perch among rock music's A-listers. Their follow-up effort, *Open Up and Say... Ahh!*, would cement their position, and prove to be their biggest-selling album

A hugely popular live act, Poison were now firing on all cylinders. Nowhere is this more evident than on 'Every Rose Has Its Thorn', their only US Number One (which also managed to reach Number 13 in the UK). Four more singles followed, including two US Top Ten hits: 'Nothin' But A Good Time', and a cover of an unlikely song, Loggins & Messina's 1972 hit 'Your Mama Don't Dance'.

Packed with memorable riffs and powerful hooks *Open Up And Say... Ahh* represented a band at its best. A huge success in terms of sales, the album peaked at Number Two on the *Billboard* Top 200; though it fared less well in the UK, where it only managed to reach Number 23.

Number One singles: US: Every Rose Has Its Thorn

Grammy awards: None

Label: US: Capitol; UK: Music for Nations

Recorded in: Los Angeles, USA

Personnel:
Bret Michaels
C C Devill
Bobby Dal
Rikki Rocket
John Purdell

Producers:
Tom Werman

1 Love On The Rocks (3:34)
2 Nothin' But A Good Time (3:45)
3 Back To The Rocking Horse (3:56)
4 Good Love (2:52)
5 Tearin' Down The Walls (3:52)
6 Look But You Can't Touch (3:26)
7 Fallen Angel (3:58)
8 Every Rose Has Its Thorn (4:20)
9 Your Mama Don't Dance (3:01)
10 Bad To Be Good (4:04)

Total album length: 37 minutes

POISON

Open Up and Say... Ahh!

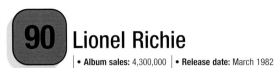

90 Lionel Richie

| • Album sales: 4,300,000 | • Release date: March 1982 |

Lionel Richie's pending departure from The Commodores was clearly signalled by 'Endless Love', the theme song from the Brooke Shields romance. A Number One hit in the US, Richie composed the song and sang it as duet with Diana Ross. It fared better than any of the group's own singles and, unsurprisingly, was adopted as one of the templates on which to build his solo career, which was launched with this eponymous album.

The ballad 'Truly', which topped the US singles chart (and reached Number Six in the UK), continued to lay the foundation for Richie's new home in easy-listening territory. The equally impressive 'My Love', another Number One US single, consolidated his status.

Ballads aside, *Lionel Richie* was packed with infectious dance and catchy pop, including the bright and breezy 'You Are', yet another Number One US single. As the Commodores continued without him, Richie continued his relationship with producer James Anthony Carmichael. Together they fashioned a smooth, seamless album that favoured Richie's easy singing style better than any of his previous ensemble work.

Number One singles:
None

Grammy awards:
Best male pop vocal
performance

Label: US & UK: Motown

Recorded in: N/A

Producers:
Lionel Richie
James Anthony Carmichael

Personnel:
Lionel Richie
Jimmy Connors
Deborah Thomas
David Cochrane
Darrell Jones
Richie Zito
Tim May
Fred Tackett
Richard Marx
Michael Baddicker
Ndugu East
Paul Jackson Jr
MC Rob
Joe Walsh
Various other personnel

1 Serves You Right (5:14)
2 Wandering Stranger (5:38)
3 Tell Me (5:32)
4 My Love (4:08)
5 Round And Round (4:57)
6 Truly (3:26)
7 You Are (5:05)
8 You Mean More To Me (3:08)
9 Just Put Some Love In Your Heart (1:27)

Total album length: 38 minutes

Lionel Richie

Lionel Richie

| • **Album sales:** 4,600,000 | • **Release date:** November 1985 |

Once a fashion student at St Martin's College of Art in London, England, Sade Adu developed a highly personalised silky smooth soul style which, by the time *Promise* arrived, had been honed to perfection. If 'Smooth Operator' was Sade's calling card on the debut album *Diamond Life*, on *Promise* it was surpassed with 'The Sweetest Taboo'. The song seemed to sum up Sade's fragile, yet noble charm, and remained on the *Billboard* Hot 100 for six months.

Sade Adu scored another big hit with the light dance funk of the single 'Never As Good As The First Time'. Even though there were no more singles from the album a number of tracks –

principally 'Tar Baby' and 'Is It A Crime' – became radio turntable favourites, thus keeping the profile of the album high irrespective of chart action. In place at all times on *Promise* is Sade's signature singing style; cool yet intense, showing emotion without any unnecessary emoting. Her no frills, at times almost dead-pan, approach nevertheless earned her legions of fans and she exemplified everything that was hip in a jazz-soul style. Hard to think now that when Sade was first launched on to the music scene by Epic that they felt obliged to point out that her name was pronounced 'shar-day'.

Number One singles:
None

Grammy awards:
None

Label: US: Portrait;
UK: Epic

Recorded in: Willesden, Germany; Miraval, France

Personnel:
Sade Adu
Stuart Matthewman
Andrew Hale
Paul S. Denman

Producers:
Robin Miller
Ben Rogan
Mike Pela
Sade Adu

1 Is It A Crime (6:22)
2 The Sweetest Taboo (4:38)
3 War Of The Hearts (6:49)
4 You're Not The Man (5:11)
5 Jezebel (5:31)
6 Mr. Wrong (2:53)
7 Punch Drunk (5:27)
8 Never As Good As The First Time (5:01)
9 Fear (4:11)
10 Tar Baby (4:20)
11 Maureen (4:21)

Total album length: 54 minutes

Sade

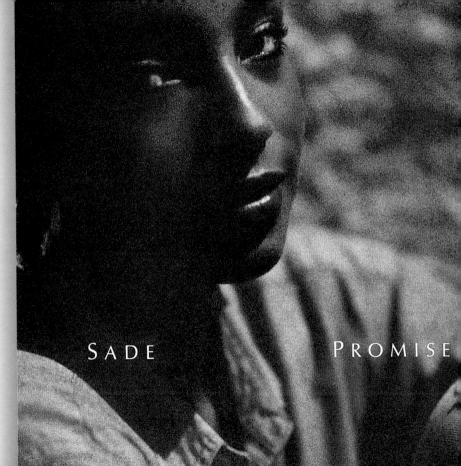

SADE   PROMISE

88 Dancing On The Ceiling

| • **Album sales:** 4.600,000 | • **Release date:** August 1985 |

His third album as a solo artist, *Dancing On The Ceiling*, may not have had the stand-out tracks, such as 'All Night Long (All Night)', that its predecessors boasted, but it was nevertheless a highly consistent, high quality affair. The album was originally to be titled *Say You, Say Me* after the 1985 Academy Award-winning song recorded for the *White Nights* movie, but not included on the original soundtrack. However, time drifted by and the title was changed to announce an upcoming hit rather than one that had already had its day.

As ever the hits were there. 'Ballerina Girl' and 'Love Will Conquer All' were Number One hits in the US, although 'Se La' was the first Richie solo single to fail to reach the Top 40.

By now Richie was the undisputed king of sentimental ballads. That said, there is a generous helping of dance on offer on *Dancing On The Ceiling*, including the title track, which was a Number Two song on the US singles chart.

Number One singles:
US: Say You, Say Me

Grammy awards: None

Label: US & UK: Motown

Recorded in: Nashville & Woodenville, USA

Personnel:
Lionel Richie
Narada Michael Walden
Carlos Rios
Tim May
Eric Clapton
David Cochrane
Vernon 'Ice' Black
Steve Lukather
John Barnes
Greg Phillinganes
Michael Lang
Neil Larson
Michael Boddicker
Preston Glass
Corey Lerios
Neil Steubenhaus
Nathan East
Joseph Chemay
Abraham Laboriel
Randy Jackson
John Robinson
Paul Leim
Paulinho Da Costa
Sheila E

Producers:
Lionel Richie
James Anthony Carmichael
Narada Michael Walden

1 **Dancing On The Ceiling** (4:35)
2 **Se La** (5:51)
3 **Ballerina Girl** (3:38)
4 **Don't Stop** (8:07)
5 **Deep River Woman** (4:39)
6 **Love Will Conquer All** (5:43)
7 **Tonight Will Be Alright** (5:10)
8 **Say You, Say Me** (4:03)
9 **Night Train** (Smooth Alligator) (4:58)

Total album length: 47 minutes

LIONEL RICHIE

DANCING ON THE CEILING

INCLUDES
THE HIT SINGLES
SAY YOU, SAY ME
DANCING ON
THE CEILING

Sleeve artwork by Johnny Lee and Aaron Rapoport

87 Colour By Numbers

| • **Album sales:** 4,900,000 | • **Release date:** November 1983 |

Culture Club front man Boy George was the celebrity who provoked the tabloid press into coining the phrase 'gender bender'. His capacity for headline grabbing was matched by his considerable talent as a vocalist and songwriter. Many predicted that Culture Club and George would be a flash in the pan, but this, their second album, silenced the doubters as it bettered its predecessor in both the US and the band's native UK.

Any doubts about the band's ability to knock out a string of top tunes were dispelled by the highly infectious and globally successful pop of 'Karma Chameleon' and 'Church Of The Poison Mind'. A flow of four hit singles – five outside the US – coupled with George's full-on love affair with the media (not to mention Culture Club's almost non-stop exposure on MTV), ensured that *Colour By Numbers* enjoyed chart success for most of the year.

In addition to the regular four piece line-up, the album saw the introduction of vocalist Helen Terry, whose impressive work excellently complements George's own vocals and adds considerable drama to the whole project.

Culture Club were never more sure than on this album, cruising effortlessly between pop, white soul and the majestic power balladry of the closing track 'Victims'.

Number One singles:
US & UK: Karma Chameleon

Grammy awards: None

Label: US & UK: Virgin

Recorded in: N/A

Producer:
Steve Levine

Personnel:
Boy George
Roy Hay
Mikey Craig
Jon Moss
Julian Lindsay
Kenneth McGregor
Terry Bailey
Phil Pickett
Steve Grainger
Helen Terry
Jermaine Stewart

1 Karma Chameleon (4:12)
2 It's A Miracle (3:25)
3 Black Money (5:19)
4 Changing Every Day (3:17)
5 That's The Way (I'm Only Trying to Help) (2:46)
6 Church Of The Poison Mind (3:30)
7 Miss Me Blind (4:29)
8 Mister Man (3:36)
9 Stormkeeper (2:49)
10 Victims (4:53)

Total album length: 38 minutes

Culture Club

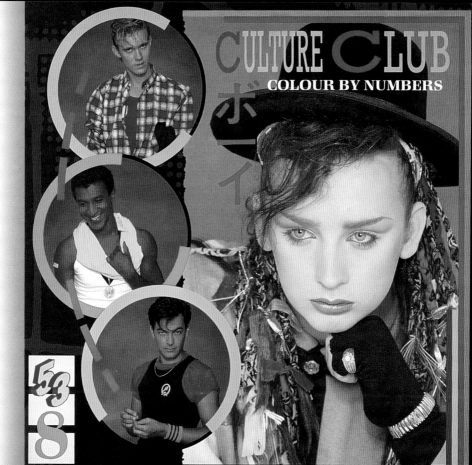

CULTURE CLUB

COLOUR BY NUMBERS

86 Private Dancer

| • Album sales: 4,900,000 | • Release date: November 1984 |

Tina Turner is possibly unique in the annals of modern music, not simply for making a comeback, but for completely reinventing herself against all the odds in middle age to return as a global rock star. *Private Dancer* was her return ticket. After ending her troubled relationship with her personal and musical partner, Ike Turner, and vanishing briefly into cabaret hell, in her mid-40s Tina came smashing back into the front line of music with a remarkably assured offering.

Arguably the strongest album of Turner's entire career, it produced three huge hits including the now standard 'What's Love Got To Do With It', a massive Number One in the US and Top Three hit in the UK. The project's musicians, including guitar maestro Jeff Beck and Heaven 17 technocrat Martyn Ware, were all top notch. Dire Straits' Mark Knopfler provided the title track, a poignant summary of a stripper's life. Elsewhere, the song writing talents of David Bowie, Al Green, Chinn and Chapman and Paul McCartney were enlisted.

Turner may have developed a little sophistication, but she still liked to belt it out and on that front *Private Dancer* delivered the goods and made her a household name again.

Number One singles:
US: What's Love Got To Do With It

Grammy awards: Record of the year; Best female pop vocal performance; Best female rock vcal performance

Label: US & UK: Capitol

Recorded in: N/A

Personnel:
Tina Turner
Jeff Beck
Martyn Ware
Mark Knopfler
Ray Russell
David Walker
Gary Barnacle
Joe Sample
Greg Walsh
Various other personnel

Producers:
Rupert Hine
Terry Britten
Joe Sample
Wilton Felder
Ndugu Chancler

1 I Might Have Been Queen (4:10)
2 What's Love Got To Do With It (3:49)
3 Show Some Respect (3:18)
4 I Can't Stand The Rain (3:41)
5 Private Dancer (7:11)
6 Let's Stay Together (5:16)
7 Better Be Good To Me (5:10)
8 Steel Claw (3:48)
9 Help! (4:30)
10 1984 (3:09)

Total album length: 44 minutes

Tina TURNER

Private Dancer

85 Reckless

• Album sales: 4,900,000 | **• Release date:** February 1985 |

Bryan Adams was at the vanguard of melodic rock and *Reckless*, though not his best seller, probably best sums up his mastery of the style. At a time when synthesizers were dominating the charts, Adams stuck to his guns (and guitars) and delivered a platter of classic rock songs.

Tough but tuneful was the name of the game as the first single from the album 'Run To You' ably demonstrated, striking a resonant chord with rockers and popsters alike. Adams and co-writer Jim Vallance put their names to a wealth of powerful rockers, most notably the beefy ballad 'Heaven', which reached Number One in the US and Number 38 in the UK. The anthem-like

'Summer Of '69' was also a hit, as was the Vancouverite's memorable duet with Tina Turner, 'It's Only Love'. *Reckless* was – and still is – both radio and stadium friendly, a combination that earned the Canadian rocker legions of fans.

Bryan Adams was master of his art. It was still a few years before he would round the corner into the 1990s to discover mainstream mega-stardom courtesy of '(Everything I Do) I Do It For You' from the *Robin Hood: Prince of Thieves* soundtrack. Until then, he was creating straight ahead solid rock by which he will be remembered for years to come.

Number One singles:
US: Heaven

Grammy awards: None

Label: US & UK: A&M

Recorded in: N/A

Personnel:
Bryan Adams
Tina Turner

Keith Scott
Tommy Mandel
Rob Sabino
Dave Taylor
Rob Sabino
Mickey Curry
Steve Smith
Jim Vallance
Various other personnel

Producer:
Bob Clearmountain

1 **One Night Love Affair** (4:34)
2 **She's Only Happy When She's Dancin'** (3:13)
3 **Run To You** (3:53)
4 **Heaven** (4:03)
5 **Somebody** (4:43)
6 **Summer Of '69** (3:36)
7 **Kids Wanna Rock** (2:35)
8 **It's Only Love** (3:14)
9 **Long Gone** (3:58)
10 **Ain't Gonna Cry** (4:06)

Total album length: 38 minutes

Brian Adams

BRYAN ADAMS

RECKLESS

84 Against The Wind

| • **Album sales:** 5,000,000 | • **Release date:** February 1980 |

Having established himself in the 1970s as one of America's top heartland rockers, Bob Seger settled into a more reflective mood at the dawn of the 1980s. Although the album kicks off with the up-tempo and unsubtly titled 'The Horizontal Bop', the true riches of *Against The Wind* are to be found in the slower paced, reflective material. Whilst not at the absolute vanguard of the Seger canon, *Against The Wind* is the work of a mature artist never capable of delivering second best.

The more sombre mood is set with track two 'You'll Accomp'ny Me', a Number 14 single in the US. However, it is even more notable on the title track, a paean to troubled love which provided the singer with a Top Five single. 'Against the Wind' proved to be the album's biggest hit, outselling the album's first single, 'Fire Lake', which peaked at Number Six. None of the album's singles managed to make an impression on the UK charts.

Number One singles:
None

Grammy awards: Best performance by a duo or group with vocal

Label: US & UK: Capitol

Recorded in: Alabama & Florida, USA

Personnel:
Bob Seger
Dr John
Don Henley
Pete Carr
Doug Riley
Drew Abbott
Barry Beckett
Ginger Blake
Chris Campbell
Sam Clayton
Laura Creamer
Linda Dillard
Glenn Frey
Paul Harris
Roger Hawkins
David Hood
Jimmy Johnson
Randy McCormick
Bill Payne
Alto Reed
Robin Robbins
Timothy B Schmit
Various other personnel

Producers:
Steve Melton
Bill Szymczyk
Punch Andrews

1 The Horizontal Bop (4:03)
2 You'll Accomp'ny Me (4:00)
3 Her Strut (3:51)
4 No Man's Land (3:43)
5 Long Twin Silver Line (4:18)
6 Against The Wind (5:34)
7 Good For Me (4:03)
8 Betty Lou's Gettin' Out Tonight (2:52)
9 Fire Lake (3:30)
10 Shinin' Brightly (4:30)

Total album length: 40 minutes

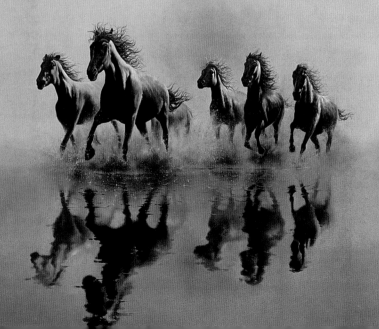

Bob Seger
The Silver Bullet Band

Sleeve artwork by Jim Warren

83 Memories

| • **Album sales:** 5,000,000 | • **Release date:** November 1981 |

This classic and clever combination of established hits, with a smattering of new recordings, proved a recipe for massive chart success for Barbra Streisand. Added to this was the presence on the project of such mainstream stalwarts as Barry Gibb, Neil Diamond, Donna Summer and Andrew Lloyd Webber, a feature that ensured keen interest from a variety of different fans.

A new recording, 'Memory' from Lloyd Webber's show *Cats*, launches the set in style, setting the tone for a collection of mainstream Broadway-tinged pop ballads.

What drew in Streisand's legions of admirers was the often subtle choice of material, on occasion avoiding out-and-out mega-hits in favour of less exposed numbers that nevertheless showed off their heroine to fine effect. Heading the pack here is her impressive take on Billy Joel's 'New York State Of Mind'.

That said, the album featured several hits. 'You Don't Bring Me Flowers', a duet with Neil Diamond, topped the US singles chart and reached Number Five in the UK. 'No More Tears (Enough Is Enough)', second duet, this time with Donna Summer, also went to Number One in the US (Number Three in the UK). 'Evergreen' had been a chart-topping US single in 1977 (Number Three in the UK).

Number One singles:
US: You Don't Bring Me Flowers; No More Tears; Evergreen

Grammy awards:
None

Label: US & UK: Columbia

Recorded in: N/A

Personnel:
Barbra Streisand
Barry Gibb
Neil Diamond
Donna Summer
Various other personnel

Producers:
Andrew Lloyd Webber
Bob Gaudio
Gary Klein
Barbra Streisand
Phil Ramone

1 Memory (Theme from *Cats*) (3:57)
2 You Don't Bring Me Flowers (3:26)
3 My Heart Belongs To Me (3:23)
4 New York State Of Mind (4:46)
5 No More Tears (Enough Is Enough) (4:44)
6 Comin' In And Out Of Your Life (4:10)
7 Evergreen (Love Theme From *A Star Is Born*) (3:07)
8 Lost Inside Of You (3:59)
9 The Love Inside (5:09)
10 The Way We Were (3:31)

Total album length: 40 minutes

Barbra Streisand

Barbra Streisand

Memories

82 Mountain Music

| • **Album sales:** 5,000,000 | • **Release date:** February 1982 |

Although billed as a country band, it is Alabama's close association with rock and pop that helped deliver them to a wider audience. With *Mountain Music*, the cross fertilisation of musical styles was distinctive and strikingly realised, creating a catchy and memorable collection of tunes.

Ranging easily from lush ballads to nifty little rockers, Alabama were at home in all the styles they broached. However, it is perhaps their balladeering that shone best on *Mountain Music*. Slow-paced, feelgood numbers such as 'You Turn Me On' and 'Close Enough To Perfect' are prime examples. Guitar rock gets a good airing on the likes of 'Never Be One' and on a sterling rendition of Creedence Clearwater Revival's 'Green River'.

Despite the varying styles, the collection has an appealing consistency, which spawned two Top 20 singles in the US. 'Feels So Right' reached Number 20, while 'Love In The First Degree' peaked at Number 15. For many fans this is the band's brightest moment, catching them while they were still in their prime.

Number One singles:
None

Grammy awards:
Best performance by a duo or group with vocal

Label: US & UK: RCA

Recorded in: N/A

Personnel:
Jeff Cook
Teddy Gentry
Mark Herndon
Randy Owen
Bruce Watkins

Larry Paxton
Walter Smith
Hayword Bishop
David Humphreys
Jerry Kroon
Mark Casstevens
Jack Eubanks
David Hanner
George Jackson
Fred Newell
Various other personnel

Producers:
Jeff Cook
Teddy Gentry
Mark Herndon
Randy Owen

1 Mountain Music (4:14)
2 Close Enough to Perfect (3:36)
3 Words At Twenty Paces (3:57)
4 Changes Comin' On (6:54)
5 Green River (2:53)
6 Take Me Down (4:58)
7 You Turn Me On (3:13)
8 Never Be One (2:48)
9 Lovin' You Is Killin' Me (3:03)
10 Gonna Have A Party (4:13)

Total album length: 39 minutes

Alabama

52

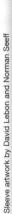

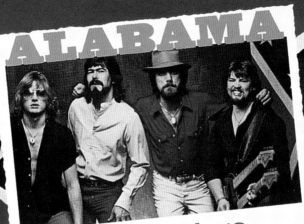

ALABAMA

MOUNTAIN MUSIC

81 American Fool

| • **Album sales:** 5,000,000 | • **Release date:** November 1982 |

One of the American electric troubadors of his era, John Cougar Mellencamp sang radio-friendly arena rock for the masses in the 1980s. After fairly forgettable previous efforts, he hit his stride with *American Fool*, delivering a clutch of memorable soft rock anthems which justifiably thrust him into the limelight.

With the stand-out, 'Jack And Diane', Mellencamp showed he was comfortable in Springsteen territory, displaying easy narrative skills in a tale of doomed teen romance in small town America. Similarly, the opener 'Hurts So Good', featured his tight, punchy band to good effect in a powerful rocker which would go on to establish itself as a minor rock 'n' roll classic. The song became one of Mellancamp's most popular, reaching Number Two on the US singles chart.

None of the rest of the album quite matched these stand-out tracks, but it was solid stuff showing that Mellencamp was honing his songwriting skills and never delivering anything less than workmanlike material. In 'Thundering Hearts' he is rocking out in storytelling mode again, 'China Girl' is a melodic pointer to some of his future work and 'Close Enough' is a great musical expression of the rock star lifestyle.

For many fans, *American Fool* is the definitive Mellencamp collection featuring, to consistently good effect, his vocal and guitar talents.

Number One singles:
US: Jack and Diane

Grammy awards:
Best male rock vocal
performance – Hurts
So Good

Label: US & UK: Riva

Recorded in: N/A

Personnel:
John Mellencamp
Larry Crane
George Perry
Mike Wanchic
Kenny Aronoff

Producers:
John Mellencamp

1 **Hurts So Good** (3:42)
2 **Jack And Diane** (4:16)
3 **Hand To Hold On To** (3:25)
4 **Danger List** (4:28)
5 **Can You Take It** (3:35)
6 **Thundering Hearts** (3:40)
7 **China Girl** (3:34)
8 **Close Enough** (3:38)
9 **Weakest Moments** (4:07)

Total album length: 34 minutes

JOHN COUGAR *American Fool*

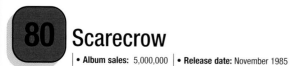

80 Scarecrow

| • **Album sales:** 5,000,000 | • **Release date:** November 1985 |

After establishing his blue collar credentials and commercial viability with 1982's *American Fool*, John Cougar Mellencamp looked to consolidate his popularity. *Uh-Huh*, released a year after *American Fool* was a swift follow-up. However, by the mid-1980s Mellencamp was looking to add critical acclaim to fame.

Scarecrow delivered the desired accolades and paved the way for further positive criticism in the years ahead. Sharper lyrics, as ever concerned with the American Way, coupled with a broader musical palette resulted in his biggest – and best received – album so far. Stand-out tracks included the top ten hits 'Lonely Ol' Night', 'Small Town' and 'R.O.C.K. In The U.S.A.'.

Being taken seriously by critics apparently encouraged him to take himself more seriously as he attached himself to just causes joining the likes of Willie Nelson and Neil Young in supporting the American farmer through Farm Aid.

The album itself embraced the now familiar themes of lost innocence, life going nowhere and, in general, the hopes and fears of small-town America. The message is served up with a lean and tough musical backdrop full of spare, catchy hooks, which make *Scarecrow* one of the stand-out mainstream rock albums of its era.

Number One singles:
None

Grammy awards: None

Label: US & UK: Riva

Recorded in: N/A

Producer:
Little Bastard

Personnel:
John Mellencamp
A Jack Wilkins
John Cascella
Kenny Aronoff
Larry Crane
Mike Wanchic
Rickie Lee Jones
Layra Mellencamp
John Cascella
Various other personnel

1   Rain On The Scarecrow
2   Grandma's Theme
3   Small Town
4   Minutes To Memories
5   Lonely Ol' Night
6   The Face Of The Nation
7   Justice And Independence '85
8   Between A Laugh And A Tear
9   Rumbleseat
10 You've Got To Stand For Somethin'
11 R.O.C.K. In The U.S.A.
12 The Kind Of Fella I Am

Total album length: 41 minutes

JOHN COUGAR MELLENCAMP
SCARECROW

79 Who Made Who

| • **Album sales:** 5,000,000 | • **Release date:** May 1986 |

An unusual album, *Who Made Who* is in fact the soundtrack to the low-profile Stephen King movie *Maximum Overdrive*. Being a retrospective, it served as a more than reasonable entrée to this Antipodean outfits' oeuvre as indicated by its rather impressive sales.

Masters of the power chord and the heavy riff, AC/DC perfected their metal craft during the seventies as a raw and raucous alternative to much of the polished AOR rock of the day. Not that there is anything casual about their approach to studio craft, as the producers here indicate. Vanda and Young (of the Easybeats, creators of the magnificent 'Friday On My Mind') delivered, as did global producer superstar 'Mutt' Lange.

In many ways the album summed up the band's career to that point, ripping into stadium favourites such as 'You Shook Me All Night Long' and 'For Those About to Rock (We Salute You)'. But the new stuff doesn't let the side down either, with the title track proving there was still power surging through the AC/DC camp.

All in all *Who Made Who* is a collection of the new and old classics and rediscovered gems – a formula that hit the mark with fans.

Number One singles:
None

Grammy awards:
None

Label: US & UK: Atlantic

Recorded in:
Various locations

Personnel:
Brian Johnson
Angus Young
Malcolm Young
Cliff Williams
Simon Wright

Producers:
Harry Vanda
George Young
Robert John 'Mutt' Lange
Angus Young
Malcolm Young

1 **Who Made Who** (3:27)
2 **You Shook Me All Night Long** (3:30)
3 **D.T.** (2:53)
4 **Sink The Pink** (4:13)
5 **Ride On** (5:51)
6 **Hells Bells** (5:12)
7 **Shake Your Foundations** (3:53)
8 **Chase The Ace** (3:01)
9 **For Those About To Rock (We Salute You)** (5:53)

Total album length: 38 minutes

AC/DC

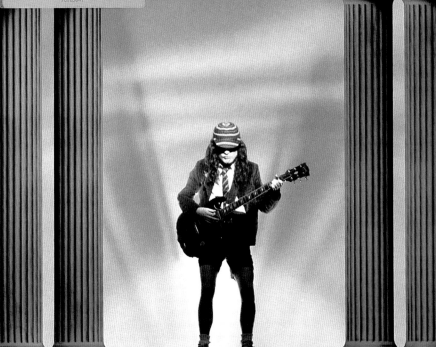

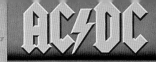

AC/DC

WHO MADE WHO

78 Nick Of Time

| **Album sales:** 5,000,000 | **Release date:** March 1989 |

After the disappointing showing of her previous album, 1986's *Nine Lives*, it was important for Bonnie Raitt, now a maturing artist, to bounce back with an attention-grabber. Seemingly forsaking her country blues roots, she teamed up with producer Don Was, thus far better known as the oddball funksters Was (Not Was). However, Raitt's intuition was spot on and the collaboration delivered a clutch of beautifully produced powerful songs, which would pave the way for her growing global stature during the 1990s.

Although made up largely of songs penned by others, including John Hiatt's 'Thing Called Love', *Nick Of Time* had a cohesive feel, brimming with imagery which supported the personality of the performer. When Raitt did contribute a song of her own, she hit the mark perfectly, especially with the bluesy 'The Road's My Middle Name'. Similarly, the title track caught her at her reflective best.

Material apart, Raitt's performance was authoritative, showing both technical control and emotional depth across a wide range of material. Raitt entered her forties in style, while enjoying huge success with *Nick Of Time*.

Number One singles:
None

Grammy awards: Album of the year; Best female rock vocal performance; Best female pop vocal performance

Label: US & UK: Capitol

Recorded in: N/A

Personnel:
Bonnie Raitt
Johnny Lee Schell

Michael Landau
Arthur Adams
J.D. Maness
Marty Grebb
Kim Wilson
Scott Thurston
Jerry Williams
Herbie Hancock
Michael Ruff
Don Was
Chuck Domanico
Hutch Hutchinson
Various other personnel

Producer:
Don Was

1 Nick Of Time (3:52)
2 Thing Called Love (3:52)
3 Love Letter (4:04)
4 Cry On My Shoulder (3:44)
5 Real Man (4:27)
6 Nobody's Girl (3:14)
7 Have A Heart (4:50)
8 Too Soon To Tell (3:45)
9 I Will Not Be Denied (4:55)
10 I Ain't Gonna Let You Break My Heart Again (2:38)
11 The Road's My Middle Name (3:31)

Total album length: 43 minutes

BONNIE RAITT

NICK
OF
TIME

77 The River

| • Album sales: 5,100,000 | • Release date: October 1980 |

Bruce Springsteen's *The River* was originally intended to be a single album entitled *The Ties That Bind*, but after recording ten songs he decided to carry on and make the record a double album. After 16 months in the studio, *The River* was released. The album is now seen as one of his finest achievements.

As with his previous album, *Darkness On The Edge Of Town*, Springsteen homed in on the lives of America's working class. The album had two distinct moods: the first disc featured predominantly upbeat songs, such as 'Sherry Darling' and the hit single 'Hungry Heart'.

However, the closing title track, with its bittersweet memories of happier times, gave an indication of what was to follow.

The second record was darker in tone, although Springsteen still manages to up the tempo with tracks like 'I'm A Rocker' and 'Cadillac Ranch'.

An instant classic, *The River* went to Number One on the *Billboard* Hot 100 and reached Number Two in the UK.

The album also provided Springsteen with his first US hit singles. 'Hungry Heart' reached Number Five, while 'Fade Away' peaked at Number 20. Neither song managed to make an impression on the UK chart.

Number One singles:
None

Grammy awards:
None

Label: US: Columbia;
UK: CBS

Recorded in: N/A

Personnel:
Bruce Springsteen
Clem Clemons
Stevie Van Zandt
Danny Federici
Roy Bitten
Garry Talent
Max Weinburg

Producers:
Bruce Springsteen,
Jon Landau
Steve Van Zandt

1 The Ties That Bind (3:34)
2 Sherry Darling (4:03)
3 Jackson Cage (3:04)
4 Two Hearts (2:46)
5 Independence Day (4:50)
6 Hungry Heart (3:19)
7 Out In The Street (4:17)
8 Crush On You (3:10)
9 You Can Look (But You Better Not Touch) (2:37)
10 I Wanna Marry You (3:30)
11 The River (5:01)
12 Point Blank (6:06)
13 Cadillac Ranch (3:03)
14 I'm A Rocker (3:36)
15 Fade Away (4:46)
16 Stolen Car (3:54)
17 Ramrod (4:05)
18 The Price You Pay (5:29)
19 Drive All Night (8:33)
20 Wreck On The Highway (3:53)

Total album length: 83 minutes

Bruce Springsteen

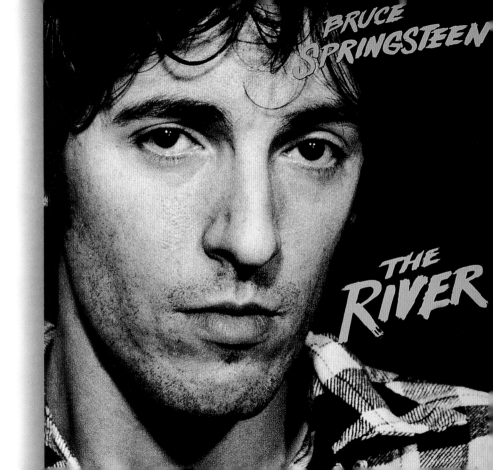

76 Flashdance

| • Album sales: 5,100,000 | • Release date: August 1983 |

Adrian Lyne's *Flashdance* was one of the 1980's biggest movie hits. The glossy tale of a lady welder who by night works as an exotic dancer proved irresistible to audiences. Instrumental to the film's success was the five million copy-selling soundtrack and the Oscar-winning, Georgio Moroder-penned anthem 'What A Feeling', sung with large-lunged fervour by Irene Cara. The concept of a soundtrack album that didn't actually feature any of the film's incidental score was still an unusual one, but both *Saturday Night Fever* and *Fame* had proved that a carefully chosen selection of pop songs could resonate with a film's fans far better than an instrumental score.

The other nine tracks on the album didn't really veer much in style from the pounding synth-pop sound of 'What A Feeling'. Michael Sembello's 'Maniac' proved a huge Number One hit in its own right, securing the film another Best Song Academy Award nomination.

Several songs found in the film didn't make the cut, but the album's world-conquering, Grammy and Oscar-winning form set a new standard for soundtrack releases.

Number one singles:
US: Flashdance... What a Feeling; Maniac

Grammy awards: Best female pop vocal performance; Best instrumental composition

Label: US & UK: Geffen

Recorded in:
Various locations

Personnel:
Irene Cara
Laura Branigan
Kim Carnes
Joe Esposito
Helen St John
Karen Kamon
Michael Sembello
Shandi
Donna Summer
Various other personnel

Producers:
Pete Bellotte
Giorgio Moroder
Keith Olsen
Phil Ramone
Michael Sembello

1 Flashdance...What A Feeling (Irene Cara) (3:53)
2 He's A Dream (Shandi) (3:28)
3 Love Theme From 'Flashdance' (Helen St John) (3:27)
4 Manhunt (Karen Kamon) (2:36)
5 Lady, Lady, Lady (Joe Esposito) (4:09)
6 Imagination (Laura Branigan) (3:35)
7 Romeo (Donna Summer) (3:13)
8 Seduce Me Tonight (Cycle V) (3:31)
9 I'll Be Here Where The Heart Is (Kim Carnes) (4:36)
10 Maniac (Michael Sembello) (4:04)

Total album length: 37 minutes

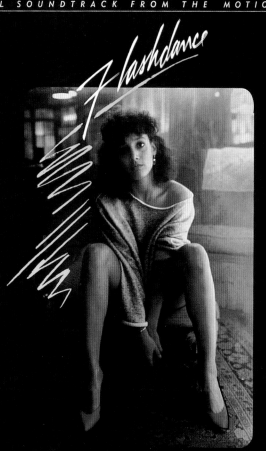

Flashdance

Heart

• **Album sales:** 5,100,000 | • **Release date:** June 1985 |

Heart's self-titled eighth album, their first for Capitol, would be their biggest selling. *Heart* established the sound that would make the band one of the most successful rock acts of the 1980s. Ron Nevision's powerful production made sure that *Heart* was a record destined for heavy rotation on the radio. For the first time in their careers, the Wilson sisters worked heavily with songwriters from outside the group. The most notable was Elton John's long-time songwriting partner Bernie Taupin; another was Holly Knight, who had given Pat Benatar a hit with 'Love Is A Battlefield' two years earlier. Another first was the addition of special guests, including Peter Wolf, Starship's Grace Slick and Mickey Thomas, Survivor's Frankie Sullivan, and Johnny Colla from Huey Lewis & the News.

Nevision was an expert at creating accessible, anthemic rock music, making *Heart* a skilful merging of 1970s guitar styles and 1980s synthesisers that appealed to both the pop and rock crowds. The album went on to sell five million copies and yielded five Top Ten singles, including 'What About Love?', 'Never' and the US-only release 'Nothin' At All'. The Taupin-penned 'These Dreams' was the band's first US Number One, allthough it only managed a more dissapointing Number 62 in the UK.

Number One singles:
US: These Dreams;
Nothin' at All

Grammy awards:
None

Label: US & UK: Capitol

Recorded in: California, USA

Producer:
Ron Nevision

Personnel:
Ann Wilson
Nancy Wilson
Howard Leese
Mark Andes
Denny Carmassi
Johnny Colla
Grace Slick
Mickey Thomas
Lynn Wilson
Peter Wolf
Holly Knight
Various other personnel

1 **If Looks Could Kill** (3:40)
2 **What About Love?** (3:40)
3 **Never** (4:04)
4 **These Dreams** (4:13)
5 **The Wolf** (4:02)
6 **All Eyes** (3:54)
7 **Nobody Home** (4:07)
8 **Nothin' At All** (4:07)
9 **What He Don't Know** (3:40)
10 **Shell Shock** (3:43)

Total album length: 39 minutes

Heart

HEART

74 Tango In The Night

| • **Album sales:** 5,100,000 | • **Release date:** April 1987 |

*T*ango In The Night was the last Fleetwood Mac studio album to feature the classic Buckingham/Nicks/Fleetwood/McVie/McVie line-up, and proved their most popular post-*Rumours* release. Lindsey Buckingham, who had begun the project as a solo album, handled the production duties with long-time associate Richard Dashut.

The album's first song, 'Big Love', provided the band with a US Number Five single (Number Nine in the UK). Even more successful was 'Little Lies', which reached Number Four in the US and Number Five in the UK. 'Seven Wonders' and 'Everywhere' provided two other US Top 20 hits. A fifth single, 'Family Man', barely managed to scrape the botton of the US Top 100 (though it

fared better in the UK, reaching Number 54).

Christine McVie's 'Little Lies' provided the band with a Number One single, while 'Big Love', 'Seven Wonders' and 'Everywhere' were all Top 30 hits.

Although, *Tango In The Night* peaked at Number Seven on the US charts in May 1987, it topped the UK chart in October of the same year, then repated the feat in May 1988.

Shortly after the album's release, Buckingham left Fleetwood Mac and was replaced by Billy Burnette and Rick Vito. He returned to tour with the band in 1996, a series of concerts captured in the DVD and CD, *The Dance*.

Number One singles:
None

Grammy awards:
None

Label: US & UK: Warner

Recorded in:
Los Angeles, USA

Personnel:
Lindsey Buckingham
Stevie Nicks
Mick Fleetwood
Christine McVie
John McVie

Producers:
Lindsey Buckingham
Richard Dashut

1 Big Love (3:37)
2 Seven Wonders (3:38)
3 Everywhere (3:41)
4 Caroline (3:50)
5 Tango In The Night (3:56)
6 Mystfied (3:06)
7 Little Lies (3:38)
8 Family Ma (4:01)
9 Welcome To The Room... Sara (3:37)
10 Isn't It Midnight (4:06)
11 When I See You Again (3:47)
12 You and I, Pt. 2 (2:40)

Total album length: 43 minutes

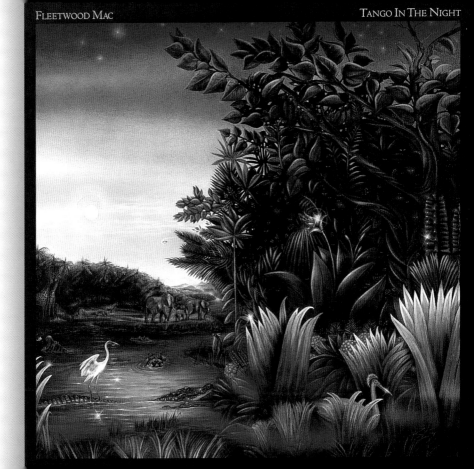

FLEETWOOD MAC

TANGO IN THE NIGHT

Permanent Vacation

| • **Album sales:** 5,100,000 • **Release date:** August 1987 |

A erosmith's ninth studio album was exactly what a comeback should be – a critical and commercial smash that arrives long after the band have been written off. The revival in fortunes began in 1986 with the surprise success of their collaboration with Run DMC on a reworking of 'Walk This Way'. The single, with reached Number Eight in the US, succeeded in attracting a new generation of fans.

For *Permanent Vacation* the band drafted in two of the decade's most notable rock songwriters, Desmond Child and Jim Vallance, ensuring that the album succeeded where their previous effort *Done With Mirrors* had failed. The result was a worldwide smash, reaching Number 11 on the *Billboard* chart and Number 37 in the UK.

The album also produced a trio of singles. 'Dude (Looks Like A Lady)', which peaked at Number 14, was supported by a memorable video. The ballad 'Angel', the first Aerosmith single to be released on CD, managed to reach Number 3. 'Rag Doll' also entered the US Top Twenty. The singles didn't fare nearly as well in the UK, where the best performer 'Dude (Looks Like A Lady)', peaked at Number 45.

Number One singles:
None

Grammy awards: None

Label: US & UK: Geffen

Recorded in:
Vancouver, Canada

Personnel:
Steven Tyler
Joe Perry
Tom Hamilton
Joey Kramer

Brad Whitford
Bruce Fairbairn
Christine Arnott
Morgan Rael
Jim Vallance
Drew Arnott
Scott Fairbairn
Tom Keenlyside
Ian Putz
Bob Rodgers
Henry Christian

Producer:
Bruce Fairbairn

1   Heart's Done Time (4:42)
2   Magic Touch (4:37)
3   Rag Doll (4:25)
4   Simoriah (3:22)
5   Dude (Looks Like A Lady) (4:25)
6   St. John (4:10)
7   Hangman Jury (5:33)
8   Girl Keeps Coming Apart (4:13)
9   Angel (5:08)
10 Permanent Vacation (4:49)
11 I'm Down (2:20)
12 The Movie (4:04)

Total album length: 52 minutes

Aerosmith

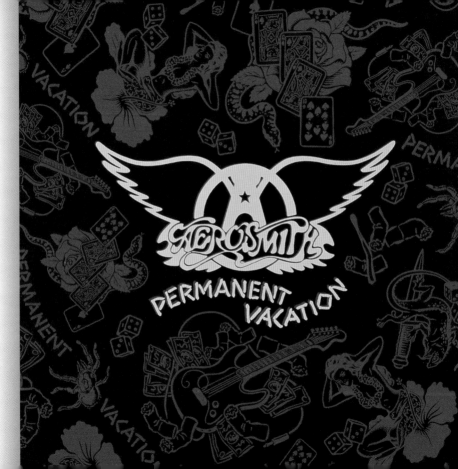

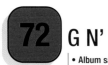

72 G N' R Lies

| • Album sales: 5,100,000 | • Release date: November 1988 |

Guns N' Roses's follow-up to *Appetite For Destruction* was not a brand new studio release, as such. A two-part EP that combined four older tracks with a quartet of new acoustic recordings, *Lies* was hurriedly released by their label Geffen to cash in on that debut album's massive popularity.

The rowdy first half was in fact a re-release of Gun N' Roses' 1986 debut EP *Live ?!*@ Like A Suicide*, which includes covers of Rose Tattoo's 'Nice Boys' and Aerosmith's 'Mama Kin' (which wasn't actually recorded live). It was the stripped-down, melodic second side that provoked the storm of controversy that dogged the band for years. 'Patience' was a sweet love song, whilst 'You're Crazy' was an acoustic reworking of the *Appetite For Destruction* favourite.

The lyrical content of 'Used To Love Her' and especially venomous 'One In A Million' divided listeners. The apparent misogyny of the former and references to 'faggots' and 'niggers' in the latter were defended by some as Axl Rose singing 'in character' (much like Eminem a decade later), but the controversy ultimately overshadowed the considerable musical merits that the album's second half offered.

Nevertheless, the album reached Number Two in the *Billboard* chart, with the 'Patience' single hitting Number Four.

Number One singles:
None

Grammy awards:
None

Label: US & UK: Geffen

Recorded in:
Los Angeles, USA

Personnel:
Axl Rose
Izzy Stradlin
Slash
Steven Adler
Duff McKagan

Producers:
Mike Clink
Niven
Axl Rose
Izzy Stradlin
Slash
Steven Adler

1 Reckless Life (3:20)
2 Nice Boys (3:03)
3 MoveTo The City (3:42)
4 Mama Kin (3:57)
5 Patience (5:56)
6 Used To Love Her (3:13)
7 You're Crazy (4:10)
8 One In A Million (6:10)

Total album length: 33 minutes

Guns N' Roses

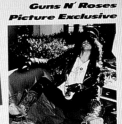

Guns N' Roses Picture Exclusive

GN'R LIES

EXCLUSIVE

December 6, 1988

The loveliest girls are always in your GN'R

● Sue's toes shot off by snatch gang

THE SEX, THE DRUGS, THE VIOLENCE,
THE SHOCKING TRUTH

USED TO LOVE ♥ HER

A joke, nothing more. Actually it's pretty self-explanatory if you ask me!

One In A
MILLION

Ever been unjustly hassled by someone with a gun and a ... Maybe you've been ... had someone at... ... stolen properly ... ... won't take no for an a... ... Been to a gas station or con... ... ience store and treated lik... ... you don't belong here by an... ... individual who can barely speak English? Hopefully not, but have you ever been

attacked by a homosexual? Had some so-called religionist try to con you out of your hard-earned cash? Have you ever been banned or censored by a relatively small group of people claiming to be a majority with self-righteous and dangerous... ... ves? This song is ... ... extremely ... ... general ... my apologies to ... ... take offense.

EXCLUSIVE

LIES ★ LIES ★ LIES

Elephant gives birth to midget

YOU'RE
CRAZY

++news++news++news++

"SEX, SEX, SEX"
is the secret behind her $6 million face

PATIENCE

Ya try to keep it, but it comes and goes—

G SIDE 1986
Reckless Life
Nice Boys
Move To The City
Mama Kin

MAN SUES EX-WIFE,
"She took my sperm without permission"

R SIDE 1988
Patience
Used To Love Her
You're Crazy
One In A Million

- I lost my home
- Snub by mates
- Work dried up

A song originally written acoustically right after the band was signed to Geffen Records, only to be transformed into rehearsal, and live, into the version heard on *Appetite*

For *Destruction*. Now it's been taken back to its original pace, though it has remained electric. None of which has been done for better or worse... only for the sake of something to do. (We do what we want.)

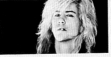

CAN AXL HELP YOU?
★ *IF YOU'VE got a problem, I'm here to help. Please write: Conspiracy, Inc., P.O. Box 67279, Los Angeles, CA 90067. You must enclose a stamped, self-addressed envelope for a confidential personal reply or one of my leaflets.*

71 Girl You Know It's True

| • **Album sales:** 5,100,000 | • **Release date:** August 1989 |

Although ostensibly fronted by the handsome dreadlocked duo of Rob Pilatus and Fabrice Morvan, Milli Vanilli was in truth nine-tenths Frank Farian, a middle-aged studio wizard who assembled this sweet but slender selection of Europop perfection in Germany. As the man who brought Boney M to a mass market in the 1970s, Farian was clearly an expert at crafting irresistible Europop classics. This album was no exception.

Released as *All Or Nothing* in Europe, the album was retitled *Girl You Know It's True* for US audiences after the lead single which peaked at Number Two on the pop charts. Three more Number Ones were to follow in the form of 'Baby Don't Forget My Number', 'Girl I'm Gonna Miss You' and 'Blame It on the Rain', a Diane Warren number. Ultimately, credit must go to Farian and his technical savvy for serving up an irresistible, if eminently disposable, package of seamlessly crafted numbers sporting giant hooks and infectious rhythms.

At the time of release male models Pilatus and Morvan were accepted at face value and when it was eventually revealed that they were simply lip-synching eye-candy, miming to Fabian's session musicians, there was outrage. Such was the controversy that the Grammy they had been awarded for Best New Act was withdrawn.

Number one singles:
US: Baby Don't Forget My Number; Blame It On The Rain; I'm Gonna Miss You

Personnel:
Charles Shaw
Johnny Davis
Brad Howell

Grammy awards: Best New Act (revoked)

Producer:
Frank Farian

Label: US & UK: Arista

Recorded in: Germany

9 Girl You Know It's True (4.12)
3 Baby Don't Forget My Number (4:16)
8 More Than You'll Ever Know (4:31)
1 Blame It On The Rain (4:26)
2 Take It As It Comes (4:14)
6 It's Your Thing (3:54)
4 Dreams To Remember (3:53)
5 All Or Nothing (3:15)
7 I'm Gonna Miss You (4:19)
10 Girl You Know It's True (NY Subway Ext. Mix) (6:27)

Total album length: 43 minutes

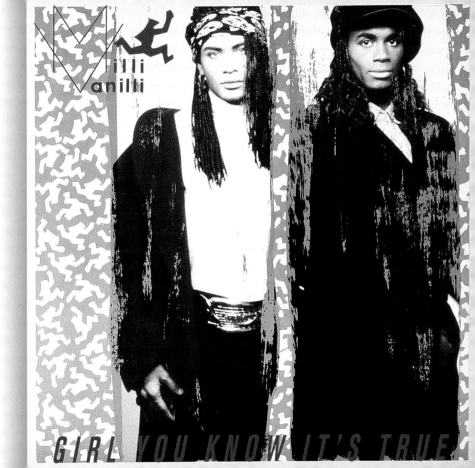

70 Full Moon Fever

| • Album sales: 5,100,000 | • Release date: April 1989 |

Technically, *Full Moon Fever* was Tom Petty's first album as a solo artist, rather than as the leader of The Heartbreakers. Some felt that this was overstating things a bit much, since there was little dramatic change in style from the jangly roots rock that Tom Petty and The Heartbreakers had explored over seven albums; what is more, Heartbreakers Benmont Tench, Howie Epstein and Mike Campbell all play on the album.

Nevertheless, *Full Moon Fever* had a commercial edge that the earlier albums lacked, and Petty's songwriting had rarely been as strong. Electric Light Orchestra's Jeff Lynne handled production duties and co-wrote seven of the 12 tracks, ensuring a smooth, radio-friendly sound that put the melodies, harmonies and Petty's voice to the front of the mix.

The album opened with the reflective Top Top hit 'Free Fallin'', which set the melancholy-yet-commercial tone of the rest of the record.

Full Moon Fever also featured guest appearances from Petty and Lynne's fellow Travelling Wilburys George Harrison and Roy Orbison (who died before the album was released). The album made Number Three on the *Billboard* Hot 100.

Number One singles:
None

Grammy awards: None

Label: US & UK: MCA

Recorded in:
Los Angeles, USA

Personnel:
Tom Petty
George Harrison

Mike Campbell
Jeff Lynne
Benmont Tench
Jim Keltner
Phil Jones
Del Shannon
Roy Orbison
Various other personnel

Producers:
Jeff Lynne
Tom Petty
Mike Cambell

1 Free Fallin' (4:14)
2 I Won't Back Down (2:56)
3 Love Is A Long Road (4:06)
4 A Face In The Crowd (3:58)
5 Runnin' Down A Dream (4:23)
6 I'll Feel A Whole Lot Better (2:47)
7 Yer So Bad (3:05)
8 Depending On You (2:47)
9 The Apartment Song (2:31)
10 Alright For Now (2:00)
11 A Mind With A Heart Of It's Own (3:29)
12 Zombie Zoo (2:56)

Total album length: 39 minutes

Tom Petty

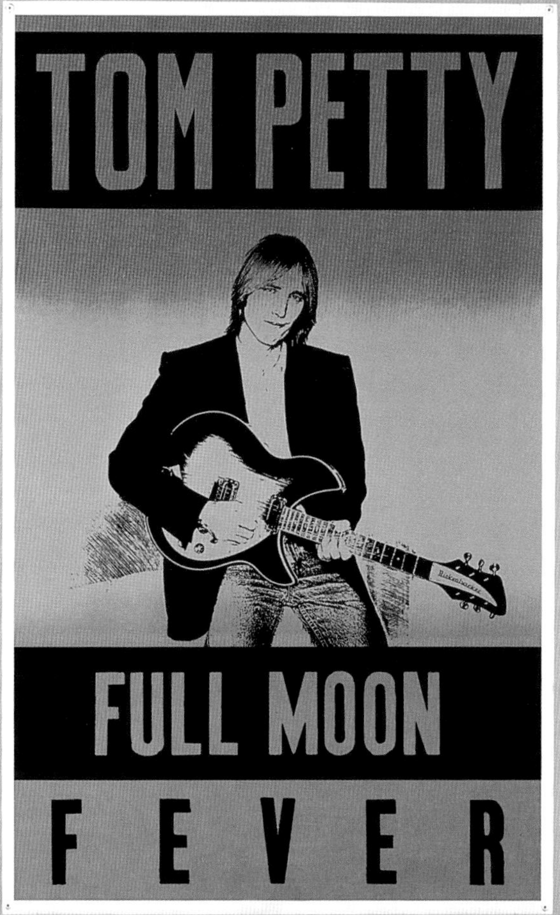
TOM PETTY
FULL MOON
FEVER

69 The End of the Innocence

| • **Album sales:** 5,100,000 | • **Release date:** June 1989 |

Released at the very end of the 1980s, Don Henley's third solo album was a reflective, melodic opus that took nearly five years to complete. Henley and his co-producers carefully constructed an album that favoured live instrumentation – acoustic and electric guitars, piano and organ – to the synth-based sounds of the former Eagles' previous solo records. Lyrically, the album touched on themes of loss and regret, both personal – 'The Heart of the Matter' – and the political, as on the title track.

The End Of The Innocence featured several high-profile guest performers, including Bruce Hornsby, (who lent his distinctive piano to the opener), Axl Rose (on 'I Will Not Go Quietly'), legendary saxophonist Wayne Shorter, Heartbreakers guitarist Mike Campbell, vocal group Take 6 and Edie Brickell. Stars-in-waiting Sheryl Crow and Melissa Etheridge also featured.

The End Of The Innocence secured Henley a Best Rock Male Vocal Grammy and produced two Top Ten singles, the title track and 'The Last Worthless Evening'. The album itself was the singer's biggest solo success and reached Number Eight in the *Billboard* chart.

Number One singles:
None

Grammy awards:
Best Male Rock Vocal Performance

Label: US & UK: Geffen

Recorded in: N/A

Personnel:
Don Henley
Bruce Hornsby
Stanley Jordan
Mike Campbell
Melissa Etheridge
Ivan Neville

Wayne Shorter
Jim Keltner
Sheryl Crow
Patty Smyth
Edie Brickell
Axl Rose
J.D. Souther
Waddy Wachtel
Steve Jordan
Various other personnel

Producers:
Don Henley
Danny Kortchmar
Bruce Hornsby
John Corey
Stan Lynch
Mike Campbell

1 The End Of The Innocence (5:16)
2 How Bad Do You Want It? (3:47)
3 I Will Not Go Quietly (5:43)
4 The Last Worthless Evening (6:03)
5 New York Minute (6:37)
6 Shangri-La (4:55)
7 Little Tin God (4:42)
8 Gimme What You Got (6:10)
9 If Dirt Were Dollars (4:34)
10 The Heart Of The Matter (5:24)

Total album length: 52 minutes

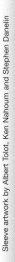

DON HENLEY

THE END OF THE INNOCENCE

Make It Big

| • **Album sales:** 5,200,000 | • **Release date:** October 1984 |

The singles that Wham's second album produced were so decade-defining that it scarcely matters that few remember the rest of the record. Andrew Ridgely may feature on the cover and may have taken a co-writing credit on the mega-hit 'Careless Whisper', but there's little doubt that this is George Michael's album. *Make It Big* was also the first album that earned the duo any money, as the move from independent label Innervision to Sony had meant giving up their royalties from their debut, *Fantastic*.

As well as writing some massively popular songs, *Make It Big* also demonstrated George Michael's love of 1960s soul and his under-rated production skills. 'Wake Me Up Before You Go-Go', the album's debut single, was the fifth Wham! Top 40 hit in the UK, and became their first Number One.

Aptly named for the US market, *Make It Big* earned the duo no less than three Number One singles – 'Wake Me Up Before You Go-Go', 'Everything She Wants' and 'Careless Whisper'. Nearly as successful, 'Freedom' peaked at Number Three. Prior to the release, the highest charting Wham! single in the US had been 'Bad Boys', which only managed to reach Number 60.

In the US, the 'Careless Whisper' single was credited to 'Wham! featuring George Michael', indicating a solo career wasn't far off.

Number One singles:
US & UK: Wake Me Up Before You Go-Go; Careless Whisper; US: Everything She Wants; UK: Freedom

Grammy awards:
None

Label: US: Columbia; UK: Epic

Recorded in: N/A

Personnel:
George Michael
Andrew Ridgely
David Baptiste
Hugh Burns
Dean Estes
Tommy Eyre
Colin Graham
Steve Gregory
Trevor Morrell
Andy Richards
Paul Spong

Producer:
George Michael

1 Wake Me Up Before You Go-Go (3:50)
2 Everything She Wants (5:01)
3 Heartbeat (4:42)
4 Like A Baby (4:12)
5 Freedom (5:01)
6 If You Were There (3:38)
7 Credit Card Baby (5:08)
8 Careless Whisper (6:30)

Total album length: 38 minutes

Wham!

WHAM!

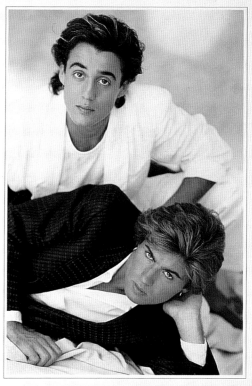

MAKE IT BIG

67 Diamond Life

| • **Album sales:** 5,200,000 | • **Release date:** July 1984 |

Sade was actually the name of the London-based band that featured Nigerian-born Helen Farosade 'Sade' Abu on lead vocals, although her talent and looks ensured that Abu's fame quickly exceeded any of her colleagues. Nevertheless, it was the skilled musicianship of the group as much as the former model's sultry looks and distinctive voice that helped *Diamond Life* spend 81 weeks on the *Billboard* Hot 100 and produce a number of hit singles.

The album's sound has as much to do with jazz as soul, the limber swing of the rhythm section matched by Stuart Matthewman's emotive saxophone on most tracks. Abu's deep, rich voice sounded likes no one else's in soul, making standard love-song lyrics sound special. The songs don't vary wildly in style, 'Hang On To Your Love' and 'Cherry Pie' have a vague funk edge, while 'Your Love Is King' is a prime slice of late-night balladry, but Robin Millar's slick production ensures a consistent, sophisticated listen.

Despite its near-immediate success in the UK, *Diamond Life* wasn't released on the other side of the Atlantic until January 1985. Sade soon found a place on the US singles charts, with 'Smooth Operator' and 'Hang On To Your Love' becoming Top Ten singles. On the back of the album's success, Sade won the Grammy Award for Best New Artist in 1986.

Number One singles:
None

Grammy awards:
Best new artist

Label: US: Portrait;
UK: Epic

Recorded in:
London, UK

Personnel:
Sade Adu
Stuart Matthewman
Andrew Hale
Paul S. Denman
Terry Bailey
Dave Early
Paul Cooke
Various other personnel

Producer:
Robin Millar

1 Smooth Operator (4:57)
2 Your Love Is King (3:41)
3 Hang On To Your Love (5:55)
4 Frankie's First Affair (4:39)
5 When Am I Going To Make A Living (3:27)
6 Cherry Pie (6:20)
7 Sally (5:23)
8 I Will Be Your Friend (4:45)
9 Why Can't We Live Together (5:28)

Total album length: 45 minutes

Sade

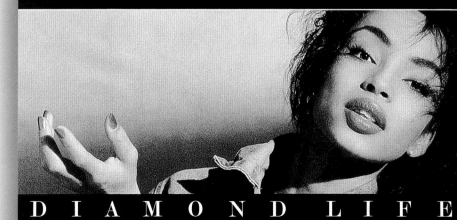

SADE

DIAMOND LIFE

Sleeve artwork by Graham Smith and Chris Roberts

66 Watermark

| • **Album sales:** 5,200,000 | • **Release date:** January 1989 |

The former Clannad singer's second solo album was an accomplished merging of new technology and traditional musical influences. Enya's lilting, predominantly Celtic voice, and the dense, multi-tracked production were showcased most famously in the UK Number One single (US Top 30) 'Orinoco Flow'. Each cut of *Watermark* displayed a care and subtlety that made the album the essential 'chill out' (long before that term existed) album of the 1980s.

The album was initially recorded in the Dublin studio of Enya's long-time associate Nicky Ryan, but many of the vocals were re-recorded in London at the mastering stage. Enya and Ryan used up to 200 vocal tracks on some songs to create the album's unique sound.

The title track and 'Miss Clare Remembers' are delicate piano pieces; 'Storms In Africa' is marked by inventive drumming from Tears for Fears' Chris Hughes, while Cursum Perficio is a moody, choral piece sung in Latin.

Irish folk/rock musician Davy Spillane delivers a spectacular uilleann pipe solo on the penultimate track, the Gaellic hymn 'Na Laetha Gael M'Óige'. While *Watermark* never rose beyond Number 25 in the *Billboard* chart, it sold more than 5 milllion copies and has remained popular long after many of its contemporaries have been forgotten.

Number One singles:
UK: Orinoco Flow

Grammy awards: None

Label: US: Geffen;
UK: WEA

Recorded in: Dublin,
Ireland & London, UK

Personnel:
Enya
Neil Buckley
Chris Hughes
Davy Spillane

Producer:
Enya
Nicky Ryan

1 **Watermark** (2:24)
2 **Cursum Perficio** (4:06)
3 **On Your Shore** (3:59)
4 **Storms In Africa** (4:03)
5 **Exile** (4:20)
6 **Miss Clare Remembers** (1:59)
7 **Orinoco Flow** (4:25)
8 **Evening Falls** (3:46)
9 **River** (3:10)
10 **The Longships** (3:36)
11 **Na Laetha Gael M'Óige** (3:54)
12 **Storms in Africa, Pt. 2** (3:01)

Total album length: 39 minutes

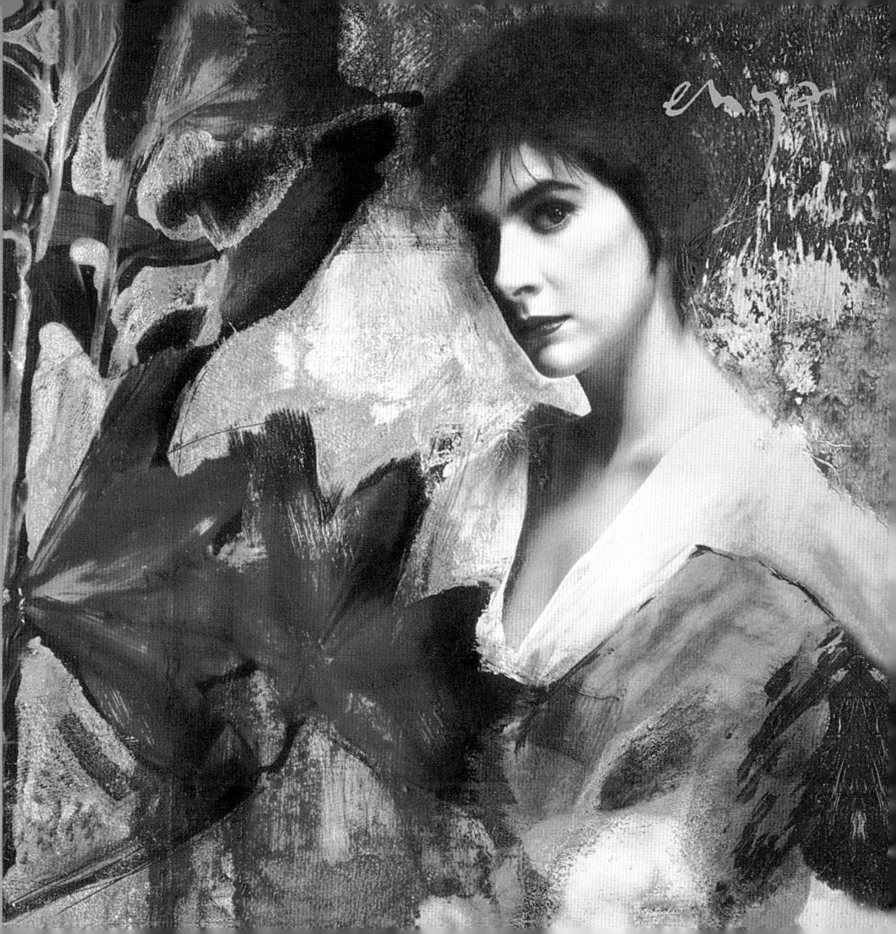

Sleeve artwork by Lawrence Dunmore and David Hiscook

65 Like A Prayer

| • **Album sales:** 5,200,000 | • **Release date:** March 1989 |

The *Like A Prayer* album showcased Madonna at the peak of her career, moving away from the more dance-orientated music of her first three albums, but still possessing an incredible grasp of pop melody and arrangement. The album will forever be associated with the controversial quasi-religious video for the title track, a song that was a US and UK Number One hit. Other videos were of equal quality, from the

Metropolis inspired 'Express Yourself' to 'Cherish', directed by Herb Ritts.

With *Like A Prayer*, Madonna moved away from hot-shot producers like 'Jellybean' Benitez and Nile Rodgers, producing much of the album herself. The lyrics also touch on more personal subjects than before – 'Till Death Do Us Part' deals with her recent divorce from Sean Penn, and 'Promise To Try' concerns her mother's death.

'Cherish', 'Express Yourself', 'Oh Father' and 'Keep It Together' were US Top 20 hits, and were only mildly less successful in the UK. Interestingly, though never released in the US, 'Dear Jessie' reached Number Five on the UK chart.

Number one singles:
US & UK: Like a Prayer

Grammy awards: None

Label: US & UK: Sire

Recorded in: Los Angeles & Minnesota, USA

Personnel:
Madonna
Prince
Patrick Leonard
Sandra Crouch
Marcos Loya
Rose Banks
Donna Delory

Richard Todd
Nadirah Ali
Andraé Crouch
Reverend Dave Boruff
Stephen Bray
Paulinho Da Costa
Lynne Fiddmont
Chuck Findley
Nikki Harris
John Roninson
Randy Jackson
Various other personnel

Producers:
Madonna
Patrick Leonard,
Stephen Bra
Prince

1 Like A Prayer (5:39)
2 Express Yourself (4:37)
3 Love Song (4:52)
4 Till Death Do Us Part (5:16)
5 Promise To Try (3:36)
6 Cherish (5:03)
7 Dear Jessie (4:20)
8 Oh Father (4:57)
9 Keep It Together (5:03)
10 Pray For Spanish Eyes (5:15)
11 Act Of Contrition (2:19)

Total album length: 51 minutes

Madonna

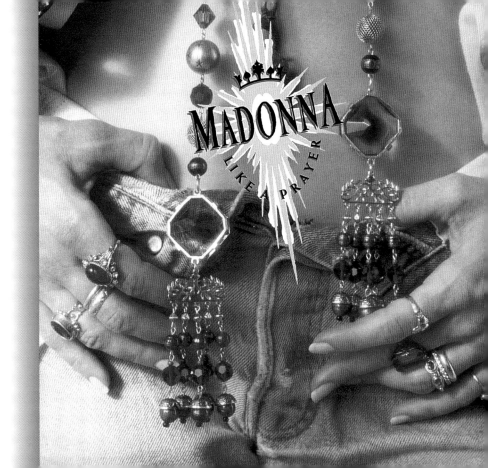

64 Christopher Cross

| • **Album sales:** 5,300,000 | • **Release date:** January 1980 |

Christopher Cross's debut album was one of the very first albums released in the 1980s and it went on to become one of the decade's biggest selling AOR hits. It also swept the board at the Grammys by scooping five awards, three of which were for the massive Number One single 'Sailing'. Cross' success in the Grammys caused controversy at the time amongst those who felt the more critically favoured Pretenders should have triumphed.

The album was released two years after Cross signed to Warner Brothers and was produced by Michael Omartian, whose credentials as one of the decade's top keyboard session players ensured the album's listener-friendly, melodic sound. Omartian's tidy production, combined with Cross' strong, emotional voice, helped make the album the biggest seller of 1980. It also featured a crack team of musicians, including guitarists Larry Carlton and Eric Johnson, Don Henley, and Michael McDonald, who featured on the number Two single 'Ride Like The Wind'.

Chistopher Cross produced two Top Ten hits in the US, 'Never Be The Same' and 'Sailing' which reached Number One. Curiously, Cross' biggest UK single was the Number Two 'Ride Like the Wind', which failed to chart in the US.

Number One singles:
US: Sailing

Grammy awards:
Record of the year –
Sailing; Album of the year;
Song of the year – Sailing;
Best new artist; Best
arrangement accompany-
ing vocalist(s) – Sailing

Label: US & UK: Warner

Recorded in: N/A

Producer:
Michael Omartian

Personnel:
Christopher Cross
Don Henley
Eric Johnson
Michael McDonald
Larry Carlton
Victor Feldman
Valerie Carter
Nicolette Larson
Rob Meurer
Stormie Omartian
Lenny Castro
Assa Drori
Chuck Findley
Jay Graydon
Chet Himes
Various other personnel

1 Say You'll Be Mine (2:53)
2 I Really Don't Know Anymore (3:49)
3 Spinning (3:59)
4 Never Be The Same (4:40)
5 Poor Shirley (4:20)
6 Ride Like The Wind (4:30)
7 The Light Is On (4:07)
8 Sailing (4:14)
9 Minstrel Gigolo (6:00)

Total album length: 39 minutes

Christopher Cross

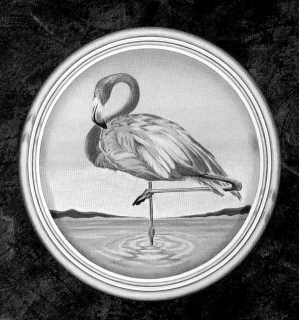

CHRISTOPHER CROSS

63 The Jazz Singer

| • **Album sales:** 5,300,000 | • **Release date:** February 1981 |

The Jazz Singer is one of the examples of a film soundtrack that is far more popular – and better remembered – than the movie itself. The 1980 film, starring Neil Diamond and Sir Laurence Olivier, was a moderately successful remake of the 1927 Al Jolson classic. However, while audiences were perhaps less than eager to see Diamond the actor, as a singer he was never more popular.

The album is a mix of radio-friendly rockers, disco pop and orchestral ballads, carried by Diamond's powerful voice. Diamond wrote or co-wrote every track but two on the album, penning six with French singing superstar Gilbert Becaud. Produced by Four Seasons' mastermind Bob Gaudio, the arrangements are extravagant and feature a rock band and the London Symphony and National Philharmonic Orchestras. The album also includes two traditional Jewish songs featured in the film – 'Adon Olom' and 'Kol Nidre/My Name Is Yusse'.

The Jazz Singer produced three Top 10 hits in the US – 'Love on the Rocks', 'America' and 'Hello Again', and received a Grammy nomination for Best Album of Original Score Written for a Motion Picture, as well as a Golden Globes nomination for 'Love on the Rocks'.

Number One singles:
None

Grammy awards: None

Label: US & UK: Capitol

Recorded in: N/A

Personnel:
Neil Diamond
Linda Press
Tom Hensley
Alan Lindgren
Richard Bennett
Doug Rhone
Reinie Press
Dennis St John

King Errisson
Vince Charles
Marilyn O'Brien
H.L. Voelker
Oren Waters
Luther Waters
Donny Gerard
Timothy Allan Bullara
Jeremy C. Lipton
Boyd H. Schlaefer
Mark H. Stevens
James Gregory Wilburn
Dale D. Morich
Yoav Steven Paskowitz
Various other personnel

Producer:
Bob Gaudio

1 **America** (4:18)
2 **Adon Olom** (0.32)
3 **You Baby** (3:01)
4 **Love On The Rocks** (3:40)
5 **Amazed And Confused** (2:53)
6 **On The Robert E. Lee** (2:03)
7 **Summerlove** (3:17)
8 **Hello Again** (4:04)
9 **Acapulco** (2:48)
10 **Hey Louise** (3:00)
11 **Songs Of Life** (3:32)
12 **Jerusalem** (3:03)
13 **Kol Nidre/My Name Is Yusse** (1:38)
14 **America** (2:22)

Total album length: 40 minutes

Neil Diamond

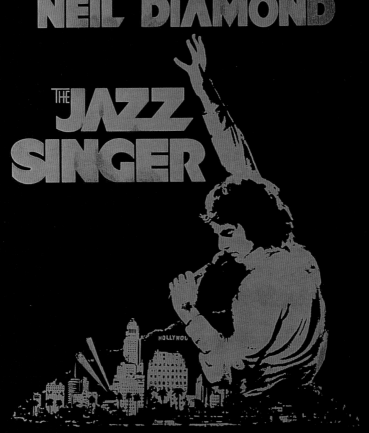

2C 070-86266

NEIL DIAMOND

THE JAZZ SINGER

HOLLYWOO

ORIGINAL SONGS FROM THE MOTION PICTURE

62 Business As Usual

| • Album sales: 5,300,000 | • Release date: March 1982 |

Men At Work were one of the biggest Australian bands of the 1980s, and offered a skewed Antipodean take on the new wave sound that had become popular in the US. *Business As Usual* was their debut and rode in on the huge success and heavy MTV rotation of first single 'Who Can It Be Now?'. The song was a *Billboard* Number One smash that was marked by Colin Hay's distinctive, heavily accented vocals and Greg Ham's honking saxophone.

The album itself, produced with the help of American Peter Mclan, hit Number One on the *Billboard* Hot 100 in November 1982. It remained in the top spot for 15 weeks, setting a new record for the longest at Number One by a debuting band. The album was ultimately deposed by the decade's most successful album, Michael Jackson's *Thriller*. The album's second single, 'Down Under', equalled its predecessor's success and became probably their best-known song. For two weeks, Men At Work sat atop the single and album charts in both the US and the UK.

Release of the band's second album, *Cargo*, was delayed for almost a year as *Business As Usual* slowly made its way down the charts. Although the sophomore effort reached Number Three in the US, and yielded the singles 'Overkill' and 'It's a Mistake', it was considered something of a disappointment. By the end of the 1980s, Men At Work were no more.

Number One singles:
US & UK: Down Under
US: Who Can It Be Now?

Grammy awards:
Best New Artist

Label: US & UK: CBS

Recorded in: N/A

Personnel:
Colin Hay
Ron Strykert
Greg Ham
Jonathan Rees
Jerry Speiser

Producer:
Peter Mclan
Colin Hay
Greg Ham

1 Who Can It Be Now? (3:25)
2 I Can See It In Your Eyes (3:32)
3 Down Under (3:45)
4 Underground (3:07)
5 Helpless Automaton (3:23)
6 People Just Love To Play With Words (3:33)
7 Be Good Johnny (3:39)
8 Touching The Untouchables (3:41)
9 Catch A Star (3:31)
10 Down By The Sea (6:53)

Total album length: 39 minutes

Men At Work

MEN AT WORK

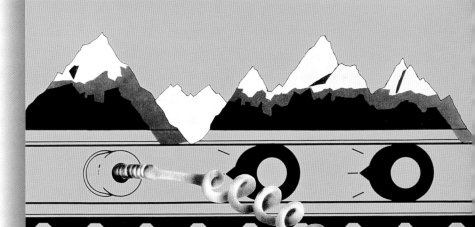

BUSINESS AS USUAL

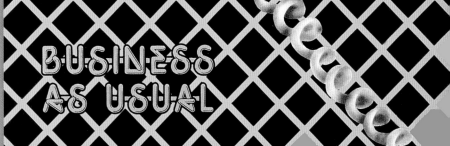

61 Madonna

| • **Album sales:** 5,300,000 | • **Release date:** July 1983 |

Nine months before the release of her eponymous first album, Madonna's first single appeared in US record stores. Although 'Everybody' was something of a club hit, it failed to dent the *Billboard* Top 100, peaking at Number 107. This quiet debut gave little hint of what was to come – the album went on to sell over five million copies, and provided Madonna with three mainstream pop hits, each more successful than the last. The second single, 'Holiday' gave the singer a Number 16 hit in the US (Number Six in the UK), while both 'Borderline' and 'Lucky Star' reached the Top Ten.

Madonna recorded with a trio of producers, 'Jellybean' Benitez, Mark Kamins and former jazz-fusion guitarist Reggie Lucas. Kamins had been responsible for getting the star signed to CBS, and produced 'Everybody', while Benitez helmed the joyful 'Holiday'. However, it was Lucas who was arguably most responsible for helping the star forge her early sound. He augmented the pounding drums machines and blaring synths with clipped funk guitar, giving the music a dirty edge that appealed to rock fans as well as pop lovers.

Number One singles:
None

Grammy awards: None

Label: US & UK: Sire

Recorded in:
New York, USA

Personnel:
Madonna
Reggie Lucas
Ira Siegel
Curtis Hudson
Paul Pesco
Bobby Malach
Fred Zarr
Dean Gant
Ed Walsh
Raymond Hudson
Anthony Jackson
Bashiri Johnson
Leslie Ming
Gwen Guthrie
Norma Jean Wright
Brenda White
Chrissy Faith
Tina B

Producers:
Reggie Lucas
John 'Jellybean' Benitez
Mark Kamins

1 Lucky Star (5:37)
2 Borderline (5:20)
3 Burning Up (3:45)
4 I Know It (3:47)
5 Holiday (6:10)
6 Think Of Me (4:54)
7 Physical Attraction (6:39)
8 Everybody (6:02)

Total album length: 41 minutes

Madonna

madonna
the first album

60 Afterburner

| • **Album sales:** 5,300,000 | • **Release date:** October 1985 |

The follow-up to the 9,000,000-selling *Eliminator* was a step even further from the rough-hewn boogie-rock of the 1970s ZZ Top. *Afterburner* was blues in only the loosest sense – the album was driven by synthesizers and drum machines as much as guitars. The band's unofficial fourth member, long-time producer Bill Ham, invested *Afterburner* with a slick, trebly sound perfectly suited to American radio of the mid-1980s.

As if to offset the inevitable criticism expected from ZZ Top's traditional fans, the album credits guitars, bass and drums as the only instruments on the album, but there's no doubting that it was technology of the day that made *Afterburner* the second biggest album of the band's long career. *Afterburner* hit Number Four in the *Billboard* Hot 100 and led to a Best Rock Vocal Grammy nomination. In the UK the album nearly managed to top the chart, peaking at Number Two. The album produced four Top 40 singles, including 'Sleeping Bag', which reached the Top Ten.

Taken together, *Afterburner* and *Eliminator* marked the pinnacle of ZZ Top's commercial and popular success. Such was the band's heightened profile that the Texas legislature passed a bill declaring the three members to be 'Official Texas Heroes' in 1986. In 1990, after a long hiatus, the band returned to their more traditional sound with the release of their follow-up album, *Recycler*.

Number One singles:
None

Grammy awards: None

Label: US & UK: Warner

Recorded in:
Memphis, Tennessee

Personnel:
Billy Gibbons
Dusty Hill
Frank Beard

Producer:
Bill Ham

1 Sleeping Bag (4:02)
2 Stages (3:32)
3 Woke Up With Wood (3:45)
4 Rough Boy (4:50)
5 Can't Stop Rockin' (3:01)
6 Planet Of Women (4:04)
7 I Got The Message (3:27)
8 Velcro Fly (3:29)
9 Dipping Low In The Lap of Luxury (3:11)
10 Delirious (3:41)

Total album length: 37 minutes

ZZ Top

TOP
AFTERBURNER

59 Control

| • Album sales: 5,300,000 | • Release date: March 1986 |

Janet Jackson's third album, *Control*, was a hugely important album in both giving her a blockbuster record almost on a par with brother Michael, and establishing Minneapolis duo Jimmy Jam and Terry Lewis as the decade's pre-eminent soul/dance producers. The tight, edgy urban grooves Jam and Lewis created were a perfect accompaniment to Jackson's declarations of feminine independence and responsibility, and the album's Number One position in the *Billboard* chart made the 20-year-old Jackson the youngest artist since Stevie Wonder to claim the top slot.

The opening three tracks, 'Control', 'Nasty' and 'What Have You Done For Me Lately?', were all US Top Ten singles. Each was supported by widely seen videos, but their hard dance sound demonstrate that Jam and Lewis were as interested in the dance floor as the charts and MTV. Less aggressive tracks included 'Pleasure Principle' and 'When I Think of You'. The latter reached the top of the US singles chart and was a Top Ten hit in the UK.

Number One singles:
US: When I Think Of You

Grammy awards:
None

Label: US & UK: A&M

Recorded in:
Minnesota, USA

Personnel:
Janet Jackson
Jimmy Jam
Terry Lewis
Melanie Andrews
Jerome Benton

Spencer Bernard
Roger Dumas
Jellybean Johnson
Lisa Keith
Monte Moir
Nicholas Raths
Gwendolyn Traylor
Mark Cardenas
Troy Anthony
Geoff Bouchieiz
John McClasin
Hami Wave

Producers:
Jimmy Jam
Terry Lewis
John McClasin

1 Control (5:53)
2 Nasty (4:03)
3 What Have You Done For Me Lately? (4:59)
4 You Can Be Mine (5:16)
5 The Pleasure Principle (4:58)
6 When I Think Of You (3:56)
7 He Doesn't Know I'm Alive (3:30)
8 Let's Wait Awhile (4:37)
9 Funny How Time Flies (4:28)

Total album length: 37 minutes

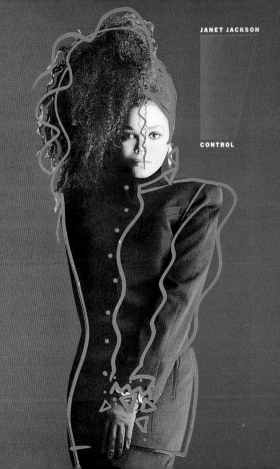

JANET JACKSON

CONTROL

58 Rapture

| • **Album sales:** 5,300,000 | • **Release date:** July 1986 |

Almost alone amongst the big soul stars of the decade, Anita Baker eschewed bombastic production and big-throated vocals for her own quiet, more subtle brand of soul. *Rapture*, her second album, was co-written and produced by former Chapter 8 colleague, Michael Powell, and proved a massive cross-over hit, appealing to pop, soul and jazz fans alike.

The album's production placed emphasis on Baker's alto, while a large cast of session musicians provided Baker with a smooth, unobtrusive backing, and the Pharoah's late saxophonist Don Myrick lent a jazzy touch.

Baker herself wrote two songs, 'Been So Long' and 'Watch Your Step' and co-wrote 'Sweet Love'. 'Caught Up In The Rapture' was a reworking of an obscure track originally recorded in 1970 by neo-classical musician Steve Kindler.

Rapture collected two Grammys in 1987, for Best Female R&B Vocal Performance and Best R&B Song ('Sweet Love'), and spawned four hit singles – 'No One in the World', 'Same Ole Love', 'Caught Up In The Rapture' and 'Sweet Love' (which hit Number Eight on the *Billboard* Hot 100).

Number One singles:
None

Grammy awards:
Best Female R&B Vocal
Performance; Best R&B
Song – Sweet Love

Label: US & UK: Atlantic

Recorded in: N/A

Personnel:
Anita Baker
Michael J Powell
Don Myrick
Vesta Williams
Jimmy Haslip
Bunny Hull
Alex Brown

Lorenzo Brown
Paul Chiten
Paulinho Da Costa
Lynn Davis
Vernon D. Fails
Lawrence Fratangelo
Sir Gant
Jim Gilstrap
Donald Griffin
Phillip Ingram
Paul Jackson Jr
Natalie Jackson
Randy Kerber
Various other personnel

Producers:
Michael J Powell
Marti Sharron
Gary Skardina

1   Sweet Love (4:26)
2   You Bring Me Joy (4:24)
3   Caught Up In The Rapture (5:07)
4   Been So Long (5:07)
5   Mystery (4:56)
6   No One In the World (4:10)
7   Same Ole Love (4:05)
8   Watch Your Step (4:54)

Total album length: 37 minutes

Rapture

ANITA BAKER

57 Songs From The Big Chair

| • Album sales: 5,900,000 | • Release date: February 1985 |

Tears For Fears always were the most ambitious of their British synth-pop peers, and *Songs From The Big Chair* proved a massively popular combination of complex arrangements, intelligent lyrics and anthemic pop songwriting. It spawned three huge, now classic singles on both sides of the Atlantic – 'Head Over Heels', 'Shout' and 'Everybody Wants To Rule The World', the latter two hitting Number One in the *Billboard* Hot 100. The album's final single, the Robert Wyatt-inspired 'I Believe' failed to chart in the US, but hit Number 23 in the UK.

Roland Orzabal takes most of the lead vocals and songwriting credits; over time Curt Smith's role in the band would become even less. The album was produced by Orzabal and Smith alongside regular members Ian Stanley and Chris Hughes, who ensure an intense, bombastic sound. The guitars and keyboards are laden with effects and Hughes' drums dominate, while most of the songs pass the five-minute mark. The quartet are the predominant musicians on the album, although there are also contributions from a variety of session players, including renowned British jazz/blues saxophonist Mel Collins.

Songs From The Big Chair ultimately sold nearly 6,000,000 copies worldwide, and reached Number One in the *Billboard* Top 100 album chart in July 1986, where it stayed for five weeks.

Number One singles:
US: Shout; Everybody Wants To Rule The World

Grammy awards: None

Label: US & UK: Mercury

Recorded in: N/A

Producers:
Chris Hughes
Ian Stanley
Roland Orzabal
Curt Smith

Personnel:
Roland Orzabal
Curt Smith
Ian Stanley
Neil Taylor
William Taylor
Mel Collins
Andy Davis
Chris Hughes
Jerry Marotta
Marilyn Davis
Annie McCaig
Sandy McLelland

1 Shout (6:35)
2 The Working Hour (6:33)
3 Everybody Wants To Rule The World (4:13)
4 Mothers Talk (5:08)
5 I Believe (4:57)
6 Broken (2:39)
7 Head Over Heels/Broken (5:24)
8 Listen (6:52)

Total album length: 56 minutes

Tears For Fears

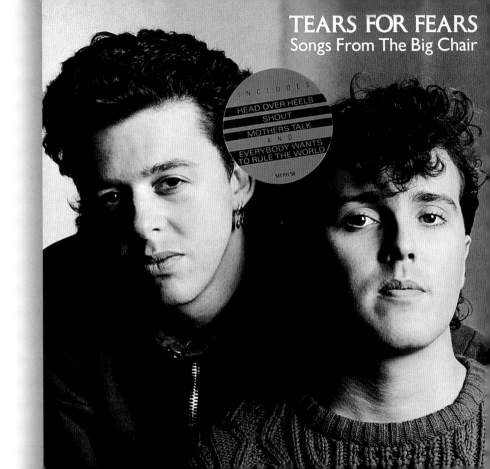

56 So

• **Album sales:** 5,9000,000 | • **Release date:** May 1986

Peter Gabriel's fifth solo outing, *So*, was the album that finally turned the ex-Genesis art-rocker with more critical than commercial success into a multi-million-selling pop star.

Like many of the decade's big albums, much of the success of *So* can be attributed to a ubiquitous music video. In this case, the ground-breaking stop animation extravaganza created for 'Sledgehammer' helped earn Gabriel his first US Number One. The song remained on the *Billboard* Hot 100 for 21 weeks and hit the Number Four position in the UK. Other singles followed, including 'In Your Eyes', 'Don't Give Up', 'Red Rain' and 'Big Time' which also found a place in the *Billboard* Top Ten.

The album is a masterclass in sophisticated pop, expertly produced by Gabriel and Daniel Lanois and packed with guests stars. Perhaps the most evident is Kate Bush, who adds her distinctive vocals to the moving duet 'Don't Give Up'. A great breakthrough in the US, the album garnered four Grammy Award nominations.

Number One singles:
US: Sledgehammer

Grammy awards:
None

Label: US: Geffen;
UK: Virgin

Recorded in:
Bath, UK

Personnel:
Peter Gabriel
Kate Bush
Laurie Anderson
Youssou N'Dour
David Rhodes
Daniel Lanois
Nile Rodgers
L. Shankar
Mark Rivera
Wayne Jackson
Don Mikelsen
Richard Tee
Simon Clark
Tony Levin
Larry Klein
Bill Laswell
Manu Katche
Jerry Marotta
Stewart Copeland
Chris Hughe
Djalma Correa
Jim Kerr

Producer:
Peter Gabriel
Daniel Lanois

1 Red Rain (5:39)
2 Sledgehammer (5:12)
3 Don't Give Up (6:33)
4 That Voice Again (4:53)
5 In Your Eyes (5:27)
6 Mercy Street (6:22)
7 Big Time (4:28)
8 We Do What We're Told (3:22)
9 This Is The Picture (Excellent Birds) (4:25)

Total album length: 45 minutes

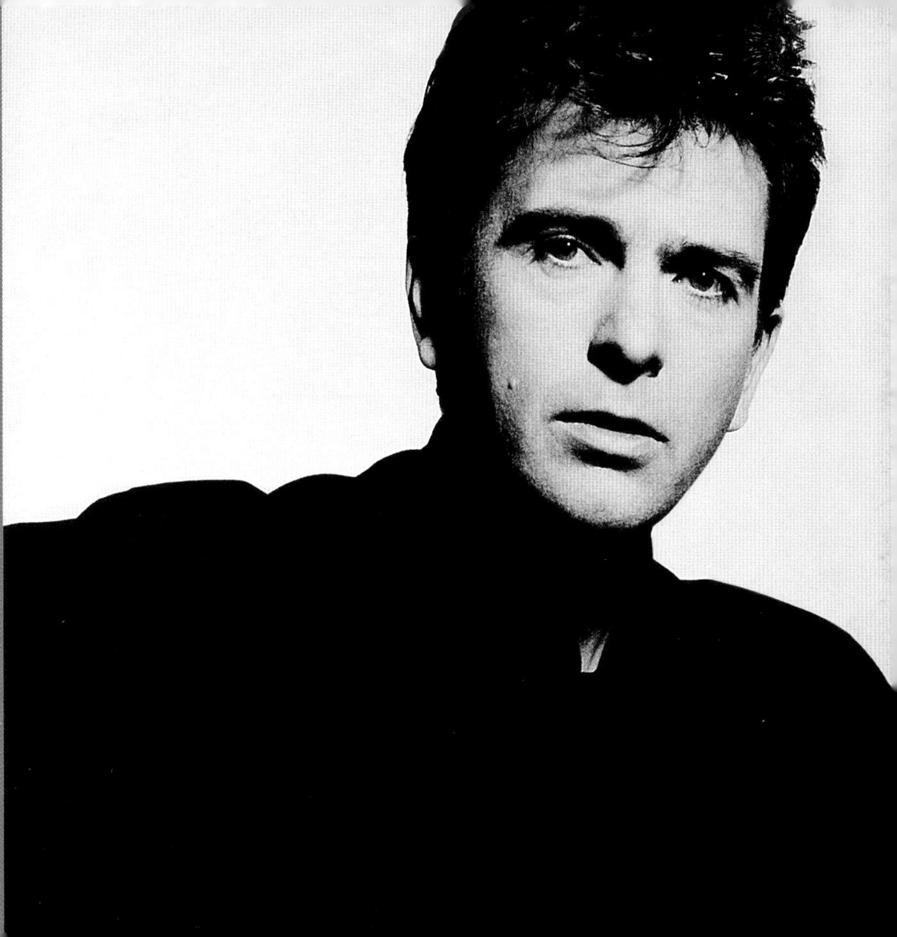

Sleeve artwork by Brett Wickens and Peter Saville

55 The Big Chill

| • **Album sales:** 6,000,000 | • **Release date:** September 1983 |

Lawrence Kasdan's *The Big Chill* was a hugely popular film amongst audiences who empathised with the group of ex-college friends reuniting as upwardly-mobile 30-somethings after the death of one of their group. This movie's backdrop was created by a mix of 1960s songs, some classics, some less well-known, ten of which ended up on the successful soundtrack album.

The Big Chill proved to be a great advert for Motown, for which the majority of the songs had been originally recorded. Although they had been available previously on dozens of compilations over the years, the associations with the Oscar-winning film help reintroduce them to a huge audience. Among the better known tracks Marvin Gaye's 'I Heard It Through the Grapevine', The Temptations' 'My Girl', Aretha Franklin's '(You Make Me Feel Like) A Natural Woman', and two Smokey Robinson songs – 'The Tracks of My Tears' and 'I Second That Emotion'.

The album proved to be such a success that the following year Motown issued a sequel, *The Big Chill: More Songs from the Original Soundtrack*.

Number One singles:	David Ruffin
None	Felix Cavaliere
	Danny Hutton
Grammy awards:	Chuck Negron
None	Cory Wells
	Gary Brooker
Label: US & UK: Motown	Various other personnel
Recorded in:	**Producers:**
Various locations	Smokey Robinson
	Al Cleveland
Personnel:	Denny Cordell
Marvin Gaye	Mike Stoller
Smokey Robinson	Jerry Wexler
Aretha Franklin	Various other producers

1 I Heard It Through The Grapevine (Marvin Gaye) (5:03)
2 My Girl (The Temptations) (2:55)
3 Good Lovin' (The Rascals) (2:28)
4 The Tracks Of My Tears (Smokey Robinson & the Miracles) (2:53)
5 Joy To The World (Three Dog Night) (3:24)
6 Ain't Too Proud To Be (The Temptations) (2:31)
7 (You Make Me Feel Like) A Natural Woman (Aretha Franklin) (2:41)
8 I Second That Emotion (Smokey Robinson & the Miracles) (2:46)
9 A Whiter Shade Of Pale (Procol Harum) (4:03)
10 Tell Him (The Exciters) (2:29)

Total album length: 31 minutes

ORIGINAL MOTION PICTURE SOUNDTRACK

I HEARD IT THROUGH THE GRAPEVINE/MARVIN GAYE · JOY TO THE WORLD/THREE DOG NIGHT · A WHITER SHADE OF PALE/PROCOL HARUM · MY GIRL/THE TEMPTATIONS · GOOD LOVIN'/THE RASCALS · THE TRACKS OF MY TEARS/SMOKEY ROBINSON & THE MIRACLES · AIN'T TOO PROUD TO BEG/THE TEMPTATIONS · (YOU MAKE ME FEEL LIKE A) NATURAL WOMAN/ARETHA FRANKLIN · I SECOND THAT EMOTION/SMOKEY ROBINSON & THE MIRACLES · TELL HIM/THE EXCITERS

THE
BIG CHILL

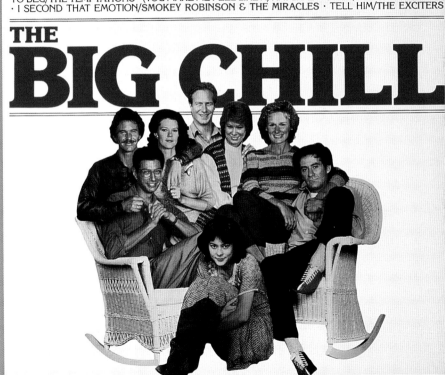

54 Frontiers

• **Album sales:** 6,000,000 | • **Release date:** February 1983

Journey's *Frontiers* was their follow-up to hit album *Escape*. Since the latter's success, the band had embarked on a heavy touring schedule, including a stint opening for The Rolling Stones. Vocalist Steve Perry had contributed to Kenny Loggins hit single 'Don't Fight it', Jonathan Cain had worked in the debut album by then-wife Talé Cain, while Steve Smith and Neal Schon recorded with Jan Hammer. As a unit, the band contributed two songs and incidental music to the high-tech Disney film *Tron*.

Owing to the band's heavy schedule, much of *Frontiers* was written on the road and recorded largely live in the studio. Like *Escape*, the album was produced by Mike Stone at Berkeley's Fantasy studios and repeated much the same guitars and keyboards, rockers and ballads formula. That said, the album moved the band even further from their progressive roots and was only held off the top slot on the *Billboard* album chart by the decade's biggest seller - Michael Jackson's *Thriller*. Nevertheless it spent nine weeks in the Number Two position, outselling its predecessor. In the US, *Frontiers* was marketed alongside a special Journey arcade game that featured the band.

As with *Escape*, the sales of *Frontiers* benefitted from the inclusion of strong hit singles. 'Seperate Ways', 'Faithfully', 'After the Fall' and 'Send Her My Love' all charted in the US.

Number One singles:
None

Grammy awards: None

Label: US: Columbia; UK: CBS

Recorded in:
California, USA

Personnel:
Steve Perry
Neal Schon
Steve Smith
Jonathan Cain
Ross Valory

Producer:
Mike 'Clay' Stone

1 Separate Ways (Worlds Apart) (5:24)
2 Send Her My Love (3:54)
3 Chain Reaction (4:21)
4 After The Fall (5:00)
5 Faithfully (4:26)
6 Edge Of The Blade (4:30)
7 Troubled Child (4:29)
8 Back Talk (3:16)
9 Frontiers (4:09)
10 Rubicon (4:18)

Total album length: 44 minutes

Journey

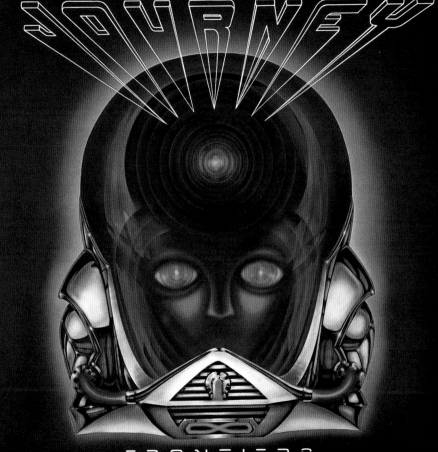

53 Metal Health

• **Album sales:** 6,000,000 • **Release date:** October 1983

Quiet Riot rode in on the popularity of their fist-pumping hit 'Cum On Feel The Noize', and in 1983 became the first heavy metal band to top the *Billboard* chart. *Metal Health* was technically the band's third album, but its predecessors only saw release in Japan. By the time they came to record *Metal Health*, the band had left Sony records and joined the small Pasha Records label.

Metal Health is in many ways a generic 1980s metal album, but there's no denying that Quiet Riot were one of the first bands to bring the sound to America's youth. The album was produced by Pasha's boss Spencer Proffer, who delivered a straight-forward, unsubtle mix that emphasised Frankie Banali's booming drums and Kevin DuBrow's sneering vocals. The songs were largely hook-laden pop-metal anthems.

A Slade cover, 'Cum On Feel The Noize' made the Top Five on the *Billboard* singles chart, while the follow-up title track reached Number 31.

The band tried to replicate their success by including two more Slade covers on *Condition Critical*, their follow-up album. One of the songs, 'Mama Weer All Crazee Now' was released as a single, but failed to crack the US Top 40.

Quiet Riot's time as a chart-topping act was short-lived, but *Metal Health* remains one of the decade's key rock releases.

Number One singles:
None

Grammy awards: None

Label: US & UK: Pasha

Recorded in:
Los Angeles, USA

Producer:
Spencer Proffer

Personnel:
Kevin DuBrow
Carlos Cavazo
Chuck Wright
Frankie Banali
Pat Regan
Rudy Sarzo
Spencer Proffer
Donna Slattery
Tuesday Knight

1 **Metal Health** (5:17)
2 **Cum On Feel The Noize** (4:50)
3 **Don't Wanna Let You Go** (4:42)
4 **Slick Black Cadillac** (4:12)
5 **Love's A Bitch** (4:13)
6 **Breathless** (3:51)
7 **Run for Cover** (3:38)
8 **Battle Axe** (1:38)
9 **Let's Get Crazy** (4:08)
10 **Thunderbird** (4:42)

Total album length: 44 minutes

QUIET RIOT

METAL HEALTH

| • **Album sales:** 6,100,000 | • **Release date:** July 1981 |

The fourth album from one of the decade's most popular rock outfits was arguably their best, taking an already popular group into the realms of the multi-platinum and giving them a ten-week run at the top of the *Billboard* album chart. It also changed the image of the band in the eyes of the public; the massive success of the single 'Waiting For A Girl Like You' meaning these hard-rockers would forever be labelled a power ballad act.

The choice of Robert John 'Mutt' Lange as producer was an inspired one - Lange had recently produced *Back In Black*, AC/DC's most successful album. His ability to combine melody and crunch suited Foreigner perfectly. The album also benefited from the support of a couple of guest performers. Legendary Motown artist Junior Walker provided saxophone on the hit 'Urgent', while British synth-whizz Thomas Dolby contributed to the radio-friendly texture of the album as a whole.

The single 'Waiting For A Girl Like You' spent ten weeks at Number Two on the US chart, and though it failed to earn top spot, it spent five months on the Top 100. In the UK, the song peaked at Number Eight. The harder-sounding 'Urgent' failed to chart in the UK, but it did provide the band with one of its biggest US hits, reaching Number Three.

Number One singles:
None

Grammy awards: None

Label: US & UK: Atlantic

Recorded in: N/A

Personnel:
Lou Gramm
Mick Jones
Rick Wills
Dennis Elliott
Junior Walker
Thomas Dolby
Ian Lloyd
Larry Fast
Michael Fonfara
Robert John 'Mutt' Lange
Bob Mayo
Hugh McCracken
Mark Rivera

Producer:
Robert John 'Mutt' Lange

1 **Night Life (3:11)**
2 **Juke Box Hero (4:29)**
3 **Break It Up (3:48)**
4 **Waiting For A Girl Like You (4:11)**
5 **Luanne (3:48)**
6 **Urgent (4:51)**
7 **I'm Gonna Win (4:18)**
8 **Woman In Black (4:42)**
9 **Girl On The Moon (3:49)**
10 **Don't Let Go (4:49)**

Total album length: 42 minutes

Foreigner

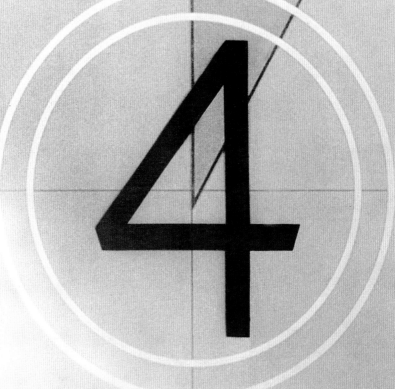

51 She's So Unusual

| • Album sales: 6,100,000 | • Release date: December 1983 |

Pop was rarely as energetic as when in Cyndi Lauper's hands, and this debut album strikes the perfect balance between sophisticated songwriting craft and youthful exuberance. It spawned two of the decade's defining singles, 'Girls Just Want To Have Fun' and the Number One smash 'Time After Time'. What's more, *She's So Unusual* made Lauper one the first artists to have her image very much defined by MTV.

The album was produced by Rick Chertoff at the Record Plant in New York, with musical assistance from his long-time associates Eric Bazilian and Rob Hyman. The three skilfully executed a mix of new wave guitar and dance synths, with Lauper's distinctive, yelping vocals featuring high in the mix.

Among the albums other successful singles were 'She Bop' and 'All Through the Night', both of which reached the US Top Ten. 'Money Changes Everything' peaked at Number 27. Lauper's cover of the Prince song, 'When You Were Mine', was also released, but failed to chart.

She's So Unusual was nominated for five Grammy awards and won Lauper the Best New Artist award at the 1984 ceremony.

Number One singles:
US: Time After Time

Grammy awards:
Best new artist

Label: US & UK: Portrait

Recorded in:
New York, USA

Personnel:
Cyndi Lauper
Eric Bazilian
Neil Jason

Rick De Fonzo
Rob Hyman
Peter Wood
Richard Termini
Anton Fig
Maeretha Stewart
Dianne Wilson
Krystal Davis
Ellie Greenwich
Jules Shear

Producer:
Rick Chertoff
William Whittman

1 Money Changes Everything (5:06)
2 Girls Just Want To Have Fun (3:58)
3 When You Were Mine (5:06)
4 Time After Time (4:03)
5 She Bop (3:51)
6 All Through The Night (4:33)
7 Witness (3:40)
8 I'll Kiss You (4:12)
9 He's So Unusual (0:45)
10 Yeah Yeah (3:18)

Total album length: 35 minutes

CYNDI LAUPER

ROBERT CLEMEN

She's So Unusual

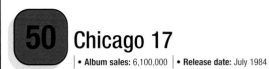

50 Chicago 17

| • Album sales: 6,100,000 | • Release date: July 1984 |

Whilst no strangers to huge album sales, Chicago had started to enjoy something of a commercial renaissance in 1982. Chicago had recently split from their old record company, and also drafted in a new writer-producer, David Foster, as well as a new member, Bill Chaplin. These changes were rewarded by healthy sales for their sixteenth album, but it was *Chicago 17* which would become their biggest release.

With the arrival of Foster, Chicago placed a renewed emphasis on the soaring power ballads fuelled by the vocals of lead singer Peter Cetera that seemed to be their speciality. The four singles released from the album, 'Stay The Night', 'Hard Habit To Break', 'You're The Inspiration' and 'Along Comes A Woman', were all ballads, and all made the top 30 in the *Billboard* Hot 100.

The album peaked at Number Four on the *Billboard* album chart and managed to reach Number 24 in the UK. However, this success had a price. Whereas the group had always prioritised its music over the contribution of any one member, *Chicago 17* had made Peter Cetera a star in his own right, and he would soon leave to pursue a solo career.

Number One singles:
None

Grammy awards: None

Label: US & UK: Warner

Recorded in: North Hollywood, Hollywood & Los Angeles, USA

Personnel:
Peter Cetera
Bill Champlin
Chris Pinnick
Robert Lamm
Lee Loughnane
James Pankow
Walt Parazaider
Danny Seraphine

Producer:
David Foster

1 Stay The Night (3:48)
2 We Can Stop The Hurtin' (4:11)
3 Hard Habit To Break (4:43)
4 Only You (3:53)
5 Remember The Feeling (4:28)
6 Along Comes A Woman (4:14)
7 You're The Inspiration (3:49)
8 Please Hold On (3:37)
9 Prima Donna (4:09)
10 Once In A Lifetime (4:12)

Total album length: 41 minutes

Chicago

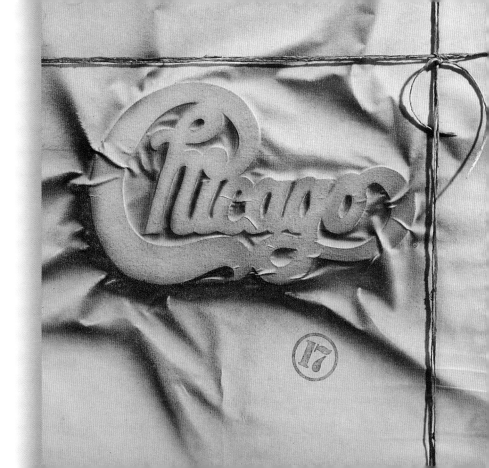

49 Master Of Puppets

| • **Album sales:** 6,100,000 | • **Release date:** February 1986 |

Metallica's genre-defining third album proved that even in this MTV-driven decade, the decision to let music and music only sell a record could work with spectacular success. The band refused to make any promotional videos, and the uncompromising nature of their music meant that airplay was pretty much non-existent. Yet *Master Of Puppets* managed to reach Number 29 on the *Billboard* chart, and became one of the biggest-selling albums of the decade.

Like its predecessor *Ride The Lightning*, *Master Of Puppets* was produced by Flemming Rasmussen. The emphasis was on slower, more brooding material and with no song under five minutes – and two over eight minutes – the record showcased the quartet's ensemble playing, in particular Lars Ulrich's powerhouse drumming and Kirk Hammett's intricate guitar playing. Early in the recording process James Hetfield broke his wrist in a skateboarding accident and James Marshall of Metal Church was enlisted to fill in on rhythm guitar while the bones healed.

'Master Of Puppets' became the first Metallica song to be released as a single. Printed in seven and 12-inch formats, it was available only as a promotional item, and is today considered something of a collector's item.

Master Of Puppets was the last album Metallica would record with Rasmussen. It was also the last to feature bassist Cliff Burton, who was killed in September 1986 when Metallica's tour bus skidded off a road in Sweden.

Number One singles:
None

Grammy awards: None

Label: US: Elektra; UK: Music for Nations

Recorded in:
Copenhagen, Denmark

Personnel:
James Hetfield
Lars Ulrich
Cliff Burton (d. 1986)
Kirk Hammett
James Marshall

Producer:
Flemming Rasmussen

1 **Battery** (5:10)
2 **Master Of Puppets** (8:38)
3 **The Thing That Should Not Be** (6:32)
4 **Welcome Home (Sanitarium)** (6:28)
5 **Disposable Heroes** (8:14)
6 **Leper Messiah** (5:38)
7 **Orion** (8:12)
8 **Damage, Inc.** (5:08)

Total album length: 54 minutes

Metallica

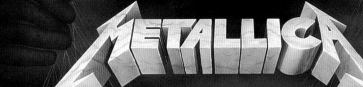

MASTER OF PUPPETS

48 Rattle And Hum

| • **Album sales:** 6,200,000 | • **Release date:** October 1988 |

The follow up to U2's hugely successful *Joshua Tree*, *Rattle And Hum* acted as a 17-track aural accompaniment to the band's feature length documentary of the same name.

As the Irish quartet were shown discovering America in the film, the *Rattle And Hum* album finds the band paying tribute to rock's rich heritage. Not only do U2 cover the Beatles' 'Helter Skelter' and the Bob Dylan classic 'All Along The Watchtower,' but they also explore American roots music, collaborating with B.B. King on 'When Love Comes To Town' and recording 'Angel Of Harlem', a tribute to Billie Holiday, in Memphis' legendary Sun Studios.

While the majority of the album was recorded live on tour, *Rattle And Hum* also contains a number of studio tracks specially written for the album, including 'Desire', which somewhat belatedly awarded U2 with their first UK Number One single. *Rattle And Hum* went to Number One in both the US and the UK.

Number one singles:
US: I Still Haven't Found What I'm Looking For; UK: Desire

Grammy awards:
Best rock performance by a duo or group with vocal – Desire

Label: US & UK: Island

Recorded In:
Various locations

Personnel:
The Edge
Bono
Adam Clayton
Larry Mullen Jr
B.B. King
Brian Eno
Tom Petty
Benmont Tench
Bob Dylan
Various other personnel

Producers:
Jimmy Iovine
Brian Eno

1 Helter Skelter (3:07)
2 Van Diemen's Land (3:05)
3 Desire (2:59)
4 Hawkmoon 269 (6:22)
5 All Along the Watchtower (4:24)
6 I Still Haven't Found What I'm Looking For (5:53)
7 Freedom for My People (0:38)
8 Silver and Gold (5:49)
9 Pride (In the Name of Love) (4:27)
10 Angel of Harlem (3:49)
11 Love Rescue Me (6:24)
12 When Love Comes To Town (4:15)
13 Heartland (5:03)
14 God, Pt. 2 (3:15)
15 The Star Spangled Banner (Jimi Hendrix) (0:43)
16 Bullet the Blue Sky (5:36)
17 All I Want Is You (6:30)

Total album length: 72 minutes

U2

RATTLE AND HUM

Sleeve artwork by Colm Henry, Bill Rubinstein and Anton Corbijn

47 Whitesnake

| • **Album sales:** 6,300,000 | • **Release date:** August 1987 |

Having built a reputation as a perennial live hard-rock outfit, Whitesnake finally hit it big with their self-titled 1987 album, having cultivated a commercially appealing blend of blues-based ballads and polished guitar hook-driven rock derived from the likes of Led Zeppelin.

David Coverdale's performance on the album's ballads and melodic pop-rock served to generate not only a multi-million selling album, but a number of international hit singles, including the remixed rock anthem 'Here I Go Again'. The single proved to be the band's biggest hit to date, reaching Number One on the US chart and Number Nine in the UK. The ballad, 'Is This Love', which peaked at Number Two in the US and Number Nine in the UK, was almost as successful. 'Still Of The Night' and 'Give Me All Your Love' were also released as singles, but failed to crack the US and UK Top 40.

Credit for much of the commercial success of *Whitesnake* lay with their popularity with MTV viewers. Whitesnake also benefited from the band's opening slot on Motley Crue's *Girls, Girls, Girls* tour. The album peaked at Number Two on the *Billboard* Top 100 chart and reached Number Eight in the UK.

Number One singles:
US: Here I Go Again

Grammy awards: None

Label: US: Geffen;
UK: EMI International

Recorded in: Toronto & Vancouver, Canada, Los Angeles, US, London, UK, & the Bahamas

Personnel:
David Coverdale
John Sykes
Neil Murray

Aynsley Dunbar
Bill Cuomo
Liza Strike
Simon Phillips
Roger Glover
Helen Chappelle
Barry St. John
DeLisle Harper
Micky Moody
Adrian Vandenberg
Don Airey
Tim Hinkley
Ron Aspery

Producers:
Keith Olsen
Mike 'Clay' Stone

1 Crying In The Rain (5:35)
2 Bad Boys (4:07)
3 Still Of The Night (6:38)
4 Here I Go Again (4:36)
5 Give Me All Your Love (3:30)
6 Is This Love (4:42)
7 Children of The Night (4:22)
8 Straight For The Heart (3:37)
9 Don't Turn Away (5:08)

Total Album length: 42 minutes

Whitesnake

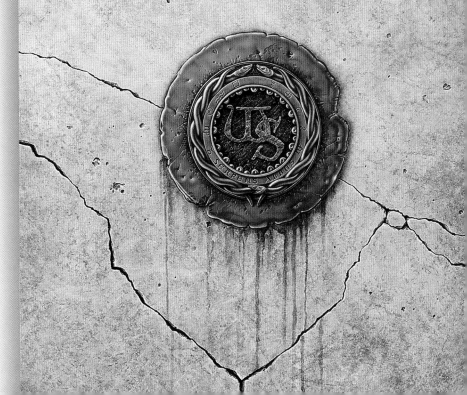

46 Rhythm Nation 1814

• Album sales: 6,300,000 **• Release date:** September 1989

For the much anticipated follow-up to the funk-pop fuelled breakthrough album *Control*, Janet Jackson surprised many by presenting an album with a sizable dose of social conscience. Tracks such as 'The Knowledge', 'State Of The World' and 'Living In The World' (a track inspired by a high school shooting) all address social or political topics. Even the '1814' in the album's title was supposed to refer to the year in which the 'Star Spangled Banner' was composed.

Along with her production team of Jimmy Jam and Terry Lewis, Jackson carved a string of hit singles, many of which, despite the ethical stance, were upbeat and romantically themed. While the three singles 'Rhythm Nation', 'Alright' and 'Come Back to Me' reached the Top Five of the *Billboard* chart. 'Miss You Much', 'Black Cat', 'Escapade', and 'Love Will Never Do (Without You)' all hit Number One. Jackson became the first artist to generate seven Top Five singles from one album.

Number One singles:
US: Miss You Much; Escapade; Black Cat; Love Will Never Do (Without You)

Grammy awards: Best Music Video, Long Form

Label:
US & UK: Breakout - A&M

Recorded In: Minnesota, USA

Personnel:
Janet Jackson
Herb Alpert
Johnny Gill
Jesse Johnson
Julie Ayer

Stephen Barnett
David Barry
Carolyn Daws
Hanley Daws
Rene Elizondo
James Greer
Steve Hodge
Peter Howard
Lisa Keith
Kathy Kienzle
Tshaye Marks
John Mclain
Shante Owens
Amy Powell
Various other personnel

Producers:
Jimmy Jam
Terry Lewis
Janet Jackson
Jelly Bean Johnson

1 Interlude: Pledge (0:47)
2 Rhythm Nation (5:31)
3 Interlude: T.V. (0:22)
4 State of the World (4:48)
5 Interlude: Race (0:05)
6 Knowledge (3:54)
7 Interlude: Let's Dance (0:03)
8 Miss You Much (4:12)
9 Interlude: Come Back Interlude (0:21)
10 Love Will Never Do (Without You) (5:50)
11 Livin' In A World (They Didn't Make) (4:41)
12 Alright (6:26)
13 Interlude: Hey Baby (0:10)
14 Escapade (4:44)
15 Interlude: No Acid (0:05)
16 Black Cat (4:50)
17 Lonely (4:59)
18 Come Back To Me (5:33)
19 Someday Is Tonight (6:00)
20 Interlude: Livin'...In Complete Darkness (1:07)

Total album length: 64 minutes

Janet Jackson

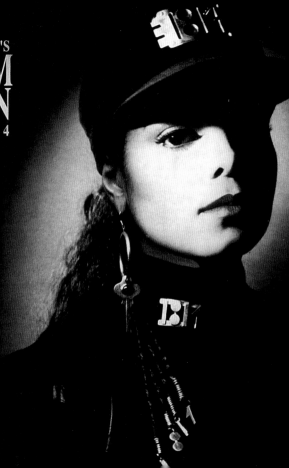

JANET JACKSON'S
RHYTHM
NATION
1 8 1 4

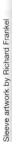

45 But Seriously

| • **Album sales:** 6,400,000 | • **Release date:** November 1989 |

Phil Collins' fourth solo album, *But Seriously* spawned four hit singles and ended a four-year hiatus in solo material. The album topped the charts on both sides of the Atlantic staying at Number One in the UK for a remarkable eight weeks. Sticking largely with the formula that made up his previous solo albums, Collins'

collaborations with Eric Clapton, Steve Winwood and David Crosby provided *But Seriously* with a more organic sound. Lyrically the album was his most earnest work to date, rife with political musings such as 'That's Just The Way It Is' and 'Another Day In Paradise', dealing with the plight of the homeless.

Among the singles, both 'Something Happened On The Way To Heaven' and 'I Wish It Would Rain Down' broke into the Top Five of the *Billboard* Hot 100 chart. In 1990, Collins won a Grammy for 'Another Day In Paradise', which had topped the US chart and had reached Number Two in the UK.

Number One singles:
US: Another Day In Paradise

Grammy awards:
Record of the year – Another Day In Paradise

Label: US: Atlantic; UK: Virgin

Recorded in: Surrey, England; Los Angeles, USA

Personnel:
Phil Collins
Stephen Bishop
Steve Winwood
Daryl Stuermer
Alex Brown
Eric Clapton
David Crosby
Nathan East
Lynn Fiddmont
Harry Kim
Marva King
Dominic Miller
Don Myrick
Pino Palladino
Louis Satterfield
Michael Davis
Maria King
Leland Sklar
Don Myrick
Harry Kim
Rhomlee
Louis Satterfield
Various other personnel

Producers:
Hugh Padgham
Phil Collins

1 Hang In Long Enough (4:44)
2 That's Just The Way It Is (5:20)
3 Do You Remember? (4:36)
4 Something Happened On The Way To Heaven (4:52)
5 Colours (8:51)
6 I Wish It Would Rain Down (5:28)
7 Another Day In Paradise (5:22)
8 Heat On The Street (3:51)
9 All Of My Life (5:36)
10 Saturday Night And Sunday Morning (1:26)
11 Father To Son (3:28)
12 Find a Way To My Heart (6:08)

Total album length: 59 minutes

Phil Collins

Phil Collins
...But Seriously

44 Face Value

| • **Album sales:** 6,500,000 | • **Release date:** February 1981 |

Phil Collins debut solo album, *Face Value*, proved to be a bigger hit than any of his releases as part of Genesis. Using a close up of his face on the cover, and bearing his soul within, *Face Value* made Collins one of the most unlikely stars of the 1980s. The launch of Collins' career coincided with the break-down of his first marriage, an emotionally tumultuous period that influenced much of *Face Value*. Collins mined his fraught emotional state on the album, producing a collection that is both stark and uplifting.

Songs ranging from the venomous 'In The Air Tonight' to the unadulterated joy of 'This Must Be Love', before closing with a cover of The Beatles' 'Tomorrow Never Knows'.

Face Value topped the UK chart in February 1981, where it stayed for three weeks. Collins nearly topped another chart when the first single, 'In The Air Tonight', peaked at Number Two in the UK. 'I Missed Again' and 'If Leaving Me Is Easy' both made the UK Top 20. *Face Value* was also received warmly in the US, where it reached Number Seven. Both 'In The Air Tonight' and 'I Missed Again' peaked at Number 19 on the *Billboard* Hot 100.

Number One singles:
None

Grammy awards: None

Label: US: Atlantic;
UK: Virgin

Recorded in:
Los Angeles, USA

Personnel:
Phil Collins
Eric Clapton
Stephen Bishop
John Giblin

Shorokav
Ronnie Scott
Alfonso Johnson
Don Myrick
Daryl Steurmer
Peter Robinson
Michael Davis
Michael Harris
Joe Partridge
Rahmlee
Various other personnel

Producers:
Phil Collins
Hugh Padgham

1   In The Air Tonight (5:32)
2   This Must Be Love (3:55)
3   Behind The Lines (3:53)
4   The Roof Is Leaking (3:16)
5   Droned (2:55)
6   Hand In Hand (5:12)
7   I Missed Again (3:41)
8   You Know What I Mean (2:33)
9   Thunder And Lightning (4:12)
10 I'm Not Moving (2:33)
11 If Leaving Me Is Easy (4:54)
12 Tomorrow Never Knows (4:46)

Total album length: 47 minutes

Phil Collins

Face Value Phil Collins

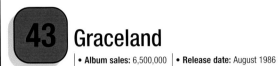

43 Graceland

| • **Album sales:** 6,500,000 | • **Release date:** August 1986 |

Paul Simon ended a three-year recording hiatus with *Graceland*, a remarkable exploration into South Africa's music and politics. Recorded in London, Los Angeles, Johannesburg and New York, the album featured artists as geographically and stylistically disparate as Ladysmith Black Mambozo, Los Lobos and the Everly Brothers.

Graceland provided Simon with his biggest-selling solo album and won him his second Grammy award for Album Of The Year. Nine of the album's 11 songs stemmed from mbaqanga, a broad style of South African pop music. *Graceland* also encompassed zydeco and conjunto-tinged rock and roll. This inventive sonic hybrid proved hugely popular propelling the album to Number One in the UK, a position it held for five weeks.

Although the album received a great deal of airplay, it produced nothing approaching a Number One hit. The biggest selling single, 'You Can Call Me Al', peaked at Number 23 in the US.

Number One singles:
None

Grammy awards:
Record of the year;
Album of the year

Label: US & UK: Warner

Recorded in: London, UK;
Los Angeles & New York,
USA; Johannesburg, SA

Personnel:
Paul Simon
Linda Ronstadt
Don Everly
Phil Everly
General M.D. Shirinda
Joseph Shabalala
Adrian Belew

Chikapa 'Ray' Phiri
Daniel Xilakazi
Demola Adepoju
Forere Motloheloa
Jonhjon Mikhalali
Alex Foster
Lenny Pickett
Jon Faddis
Randy Brecker
Lew Soloff
Alan Rubin
Michelle Cobbs
Youssou N'Dour
Cesar Rosas
David Hildago
Steve Berlin
Various other personnel

Producer:
Paul Simon

1 The Boy In The Bubble (3:59)
2 Graceland (4:50)
3 I Know What I Know (3:13)
4 Gumboots (2:44)
5 Diamonds On The Soles Of Her Shoes (5:48)
6 You Can Call Me Al (4:40)
7 Under African Skies (3:37)
8 Homeless (3:48)
9 Crazy Love, Volume II (4:18)
10 That Was Your Mother (2:52)
11 All Around The World Or The Myth Of... (5:46)

Total album length: 44 minutes

Paul Simon

PAUL · SIMON
GRACELAND

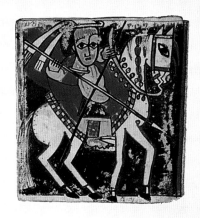

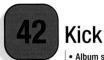

42 Kick

| • **Album sales:** 6,900,000 | • **Release date:** January 1987 |

Having teetered toward the edge of stardom during the mid-1980s Australia's INXS jumped straight into the pop super-league with 1987's *Kick*. With their achingly cool dance/rock hybrid, INXS fired off a quartet of hugely successful singles that were helped by slick MTV-friendly videos featuring frontman Michael Hutchence's good looks and leather-clad swagger.

Kick found the nine-year-old band at the peak of its career mixing an appealing sexuality with mild political leanings and an infectious and highly polished, funk-rock groove that would find them building a stadium-filling live reputation and being rated alongside pop goliaths such as REM and U2.

Along with the band's only Number One US single 'Need You Tonight', the songs 'New Sensation', 'Devil Inside' and emotive ballad 'Never Tear Us Apart' all found their way into the Top Ten on the *Billboard* singles chart. However, it wasn't the singles that made *Kick* so appealing, setting it apart from the band's previous albums, it was the distinct lack of fillers. Almost every song was of near-equal quality.

Kick became a huge multi-million-selling hit, the likes of which the band would never replicate. It peaked at Number Three on the Billboard 200.

Number One singles:
US: Need You Tonight

Grammy awards:
None

Label: US: Atlantic;
UK: Mercury

Recorded in: Paris,
France; Sydney, Australia

Personnel:
Michael Hutchence
Kirk Pengilly
Andrew Farriss
Tim Farriss
Garry Gary Beers
Jon Farriss

Producer:
Chris Thomas

1   Guns In The Sky (2:20)
2   New Sensation (3:39)
3   Devil Inside (5:11)
4   Need You Tonight (3:04)
5   Mediate (2:32)
6   The Loved One (3:25)
7   Wild Life (3:07)
8   Never Tear Us Apart (3:02)
9   Mystify (3:15)
10 Kick (3:13)
11 Calling All Nations (3:00)
12 Tiny Daggers (3:29)

Total album length: 39 minutes

INXS
★ ★ ★ ★ ★
KICK

MERH 114
INCLUDES
THE HITS
★ ★ ★ ★
NEW SENSATION
★ ★ ★ ★
NEED YOU TONIGHT
★ ★ ★ ★
DEVIL INSIDE
REMOVABLE STICKER

Sleeve artwork by Nick Egan

41 Glass Houses

| • **Album sales:** 7,100,000 | • **Release date:** March 1980 |

Having built his career on piano-based ballads, Billy Joel adopted an alternative stance on *Glass Houses*, his response to the burgeoning new wave scene. A couple of months after its release the album found its way to the peak of the American pop album chart where it stayed for six weeks.

Combining his artful talent for melodious composition with a newfound visceral passion, Joel enjoyed considerable success with a string of hit singles, beginning with 'You May Be Right', which peaked at Number Seven on the *Billboard* Hot 100. Although it only reached Number 14 in the UK, 'It's Still Rock & Roll To Me' topped the US chart, providing Joel with his first Number One single. 'Sometimes A Fantasy' and 'C'etait Toi (You Were The One)' were also released as singles, but it was 'Sleeping With The Television On', an album-only track, that received the greatest critical praise.

Although it was unlikely to have won new fans among the new wave crowd, *Glass Houses* was a brave and impressive musical change of direction, and further proved Joel's musical flexibility. It earned Joel his fifth Grammy award for Best Male Rock Vocal Performance. The album was also nominated for the Best Album Grammy, but lost out to the Christopher Cross' eponymous debut.

Number One singles:
US: It's Still Rock & Roll To Me

Grammy awards:
Best Male Rock Vocal Performance

Label: US: Columbia; UK: CBS

Recorded in: N/A

Personnel:
Billy Joel
Richie Cannata
Liberty DeVitto
Russell Javors
Doug Stegmeyer
Dave Brown

Producers:
Phil Ramone
Billy Joel

1 **You May Be Right** (4:15)
2 **Sometimes a Fantasy** (3:40)
3 **Don't Ask Me Why** (2:59)
4 **It's Still Rock & Roll to Me** (2:57)
5 **All for Leyna** (4:15)
6 **I Don't Want to Be Alone** (3:57)
7 **Sleeping With the Television On** (3:02)
8 **C'Etait Toi (You Were the One)** (3:25)
9 **Close to the Borderline** (3:47)
10 **Through the Long Night** (5:15)

Total Album length: 34 minutes

Billy Joel

BILLY JOEL

GLASS HOUSES

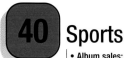
| • Album sales: 7,100,000 | • Release date: September 1983 |

Personifying the conservative sensibilities and slick-production that drove much of American pop of the 1980s, Huey Lewis & The News honed their tight bar band sound with great success on *Sports*, their third album.

The band was criticised as vacuous by some, celebrated by others as light-hearted exponents of good-time, hook-heavy, pop-orientated rock, but there is no denying that Huey Lewis & The News had a timely ability to appeal.

Originally scheduled for release in late 1982, *Sports* was held back for nearly a full year. It topped the *Billboard* Hot 100 in June 1984, and took up residence on the US charts for the next three years, during which time it retook the Number One spot on numerous occasions.

Nearly half of the album's 11 tracks became hit singles. Although none of the songs managed to top the US singles chart, 'Heart and Soul', 'I Want A New Drug', 'If This Is It' and 'The Heart Of Rock & Roll' all made the Top Ten. A fifth single, 'Walking On A Thin Line', easily managed to make it into the Top 40. Such was the popularity of Huey Lewis & The News that the band opened the 1985 Grammy awards ceremony with 'The Heart Of Rock & Roll'.

Number One singles:
None

Grammy awards: Best Music Video, Long Form – The Heart Of Rock & Roll

Label: US & UK: Chrysalis

Recorded In: Berkeley, Sausalito & San Francisco, USA

Personnel:
Huey Lewis
Bill Gibson
Mario Cipollina
Johnny Colla
Chris Hayes
Sean Hopper
John McFee

Producer:
Jim Gaines

1   The Heart Of Rock & Roll (5:01)
2   Heart And Soul (4:10)
3   Bad Is Bad (3:46)
4   I Want A New Drug (4:46)
5   Walking On A Thin Line (5:08)
6   Finally Found A Home (3:42)
7   If This Is It (3:46)
8   You Crack Me Up (3:39)
9   Honky Tonk Blues (3:16)
10 The Heart Of Rock & Roll (5:12)
11 Walking On A Thin Line (5:39)

Total album length: 37 minutes

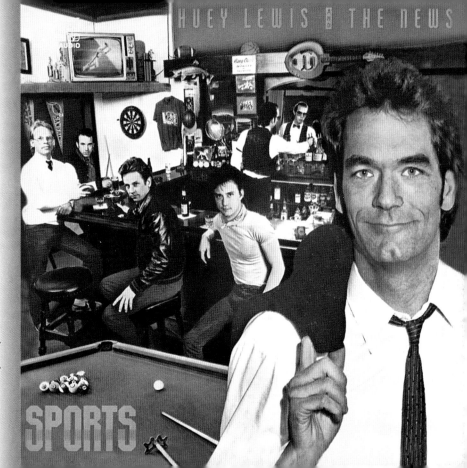

HUEY LEWIS & THE NEWS

SPORTS

39 ...And Justice For All

| • **Album sales:** 7,100,000 | • **Release date:** September 1988 |

Two years after the tragic death of bassist Cliff Burton, Metallica regrouped with Flotsam & Jetsam bassist Jason Newsted to release the double album *...And Justice For All*, which re-established their mastery of the high-speed thrash-metal genre.

Recorded at One On One Studio, Los Angeles, California, between January and May 1988, *...And Justice for All* was Metallica's most ambitious album to date in terms of composition. Amid drummer Lars Ulrich's breakneck beats and Kirk Hammett's rocket-fuelled guitar, the band did find time to experiment with guitar arpeggios, harmonised leads and changes in pace. Not least

on the single 'One', a ballad inspired by Dalton Trumbo's anti-war novel *Johnny Got His Gun*. 'One' was backed by Metallica's first video and became their first hit-single reaching Number 35 on the *Billboard* Hot 100 in 1989.

With subject matter ranging from insanity, in 'The Frayed Ends of Sanity', to injustice, on the title track, *...And Justice for All* wasn't the most attractive proposition for MTV and American commercial radio. However, it became the first Metallica album to find its way into the US Top Ten, peak peaking at Number Six. *...And Justice for All* reached Number Four in the UK, their highest position to date. In 1989, the single 'One' earned the band a Grammy award for Best Metal Performance.

Number One singles:
None

Grammy awards:
Best metal performance – One

Label: US: Elektra; UK: Vertigo

Recorded in:
Los Angeles, USA

Personnel:
James Hetfield
Kirk Hammett
Jason Newsted
Lars Ulrich

Producers:
Flemming Rasmussen
James Hetfield
Kirk Hammett
Jason Newsted
Lars Ulrich

1 **Blackened** (6:40)
2 **...And Justice For All** (9:44)
3 **Eye Of The Beholder** (6:25)
4 **One** (7:24)
5 **The Shortest Straw** (6:35)
6 **Harvester Of Sorrow** (5:42)
7 **The Frayed Ends Of Sanity** (7:40)
8 **To Live Is To Die** (9:48)
9 **Dyers Eve** (5:12)

Total album length: 65 minutes

Metallica

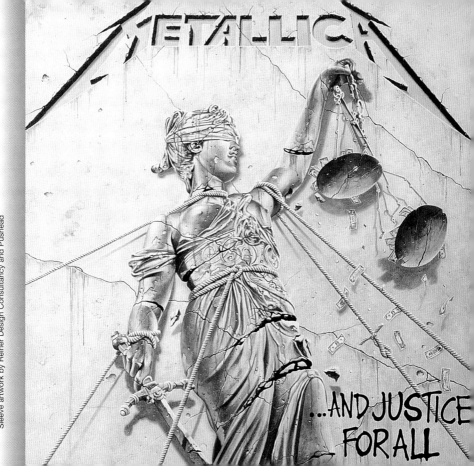

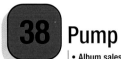

38 Pump

| • Album sales: 7,100,000 | • Release date: September 1989 |

Having staged one of the few successful comebacks in rock history with 1987's *Permanent Vacation*, Aerosmith cemented their return by continuing to embrace elements of pop on *Pump*. Unlike its predecessor, *Pump* featured relatively few external songwriters with Jim Vallance and Desmond Child being the only two supporting the band's in-house talent.

In keeping with Aerosmith's past, *Pump* overflowed with raunchy rock, blues-based rhythms and sexy subject matter. One good example is 'Love In An Elevator', which peaked at Number Five in the US and Number 13 in the UK. A more serious cut, 'Janie's Got a Gun', dealt with child abuse as its subject. Penned by Steve Tyler and Tom Hamilton, it proved a major chart success, aided by a highly cinematic video. The song reached Number Four in the US and went on to earn Aerosmith a Grammy for Best Rock Performance.

Other hits came in the way of power-ballad 'What it Takes' and the strident 'The Other Side', both US Top 40 singles.

The album rose to Number Five in the US and Number Three in the UK and was supported by an enormous international stadium tour.

Number One singles:
None

Grammy awards:
Best rock performance by a duo or group with vocal – Janies Got A Gun

Label: US & UK: Geffen

Recorded in:
Vancouver, Canada

Producer:
Bruce Fairbairn

Personnel:
Steven Tyler
Joe Perry
Brad Whitford
Tom Hamilton
Joey Kramer
Catherine Epps
John Webster
Bob Dowd
Tom Keenlyside
Ian Putz
Henry Christian
Bruce Fairbairn

1 Young Lust (4:18)
2 F.I.N.E. (4:09)
3 Going Down/Love In An Elevator (5:38)
4 Monkey On My Back (3:57)
5 Water Song/Janie's Got A Gun (5:38)
6 Dulcimer Stomp/The Other Side (4:56)
7 My Girl (3:10)
8 Don't Get Mad, Get Even (4:48)
9 Hoodoo/Voodoo Medicine Man (4:39)
10 What It Takes (6:28)

Total album length: 45 minutes

Aerosmith

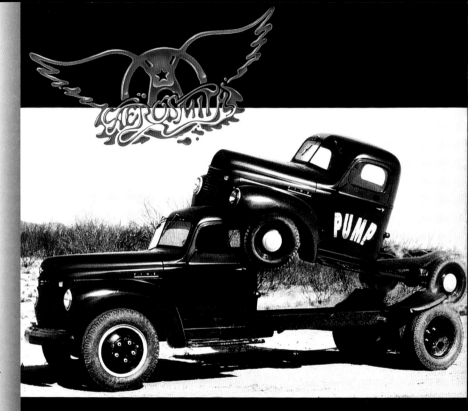

Sleeve artwork by Norman Seeff

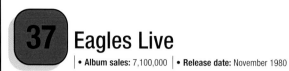

| • Album sales: 7,100,000 | • Release date: November 1980 |

Despite the huge success of their previous album, *The Long Run*, growing frustrations within the band would mean the Eagles' double-album *Eagles Live* would end up being the band's unintentional swansong.

The majority of *Eagles Live* was recorded during a series of concerts at the Forum in Los Angeles in 1976 and at the Santa Monica Civic auditorium in 1980. The result is a blend of career-spanning tracks. Alongside early songs, such as the ballad 'Desperado' and 'Take It Easy'

comes later work including 'Hotel California' and 'The Long Run', which Glenn Frey introduces as 'our tribute to Memphis, Tennessee'. The album also contains some interesting performances of songs from Joe Walsh's solo career, including 'All Night Long', from the soundtrack to the movie *Urban Cowboy*.

Eagles Live made its way to Number Five in US before going multi-platinum. The Eagles also enjoyed a minor US hit with the single, 'Seven Bridges Road', a cover of the Steve Young song.

Number One singles:
None

Grammy awards:
None

Label: US & UK: Asylum

Recorded in: Los Angeles, Santa Monica & Long Beach, USA

Personnel:
Glenn Frey
Joe Walsh
Don Felder

Timothy B Schmidt
Don Henley
Jage Jackson
Phil Kenzie
Joe Vitale
Vince Melamed
J.D. Souther
Ahlby Galuten
Randy Meisner
Bernie Leadon
David Sanborn
Jim Ed Norman

Producer:
Bill Szymczyk

1 Hotel California (6:55)
2 Heartache Tonight (4:35)
3 I Can't Tell You Why (5:24)
4 The Long Run (5:35)
5 New Kid In Town (5:45)
6 Life's Been Good (9:38)
7 Seven Bridges Road (3:25)
8 Wasted Time (5:40)
9 Take It To The Limit (5:20)
10 Doolin-Dalton (0:44)
11 Desperado (4:04)
12 Saturday Night (3:55)
13 All Night Long (5:40)
14 Life In The Fast Lane (5:10)
15 Take It Easy (5:20)

Total album length: 77 minutes

Eagles

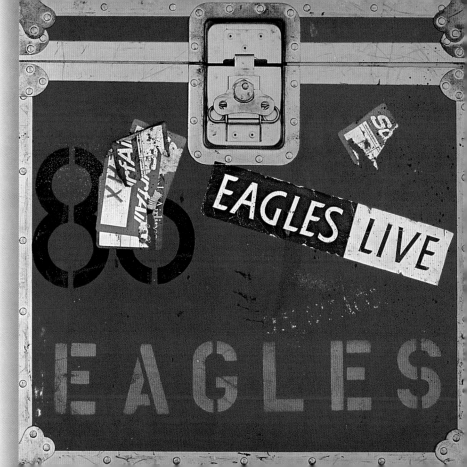

36 Invisible Touch

• Album sales: 7,200,000 **• Release date:** June 1986

Combining pop and progressive rock, *Invisible Touch* provided Genesis with their first US platinum album. Although frontman Phil Collins enjoyed a thriving solo career, guitarist Mike Rutherford was having success with his band Mike & The Mechanics, and keyboard player Tony Banks was busy recording movie scores, the English trio somehow managed to find time to support the release of *Invisible Touch* with their biggest-ever international tour.

Released in the band's twentieth year, *Invisible Touch* proved to be Genesis's most commercially successful album. Six times platinum, it spawned five US Top Five singles, and made Genesis the first band to achieve the feat. The title song provided the band with its very first US Number

One single (Number Three in the UK). Despite its eight-minute running time, 'Tonight, Tonight, Tonight' reached Number Three in the US, and peaked at Number 18 in the UK. Another single 'Land Of Confusion', commenting on the culture of greed in the 1980s, was supported by an impressive music video which used the talents of a team from Spitting Image, a satirical UK television show. The song went on to win a Grammy award for Best Concept Music Video.

Recorded at the Farm, Surrey, England, like so many Genesis albums, *Invisible Touch* peaked at Number Three in the UK. It was the band's first album since 1979's *...And then There Were Three* to fail to top the UK chart.

Number One singles:
US: Invisible Touch

Grammy awards: Best concept music video – Land Of Confusion

Label: US: Atco; UK: Virgin

Recorded in: Surrey, UK

Personnel:
Phil Collins
Mike Rutherford
Tony Banks

Producers:
Hugh Padgham
Phil Collins
Mike Rutherford
Tony Banks

1 Invisible Touch (3:26)
2 Tonight, Tonight, Tonight (8:50)
3 Land Of Confusion (4:44)
4 In Too Deep (4:57)
5 Anything She Does (4:06)
6 Domino, Pt. 1 - In the Glow of the Night... (10:41)
7 Throwing It All Away (3:48)
8 The Brazilian (4:49)

Total album length: 42 minutes

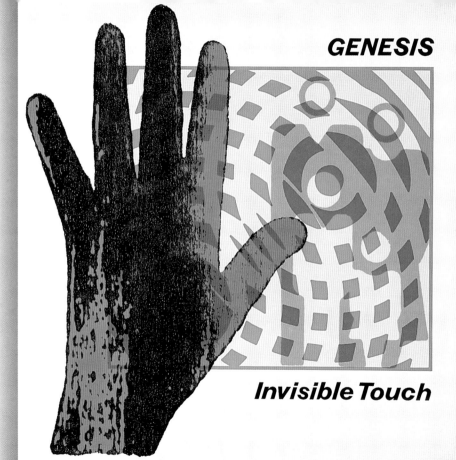

GENESIS

Invisible Touch

Sleeve artwork by Baker Dave

35 Tracy Chapman

| • **Album sales:** 7,200,000 | • **Release date:** April 1988 |

Tracy Chapman's eponymous debut was of such emotive power that it not only impacted heavily on the charts on both sides of the Atlantic, but cast the spotlight back on the art of singer-songwriting not celebrated since the 1970s.

Tracy Chapman showcased the Boston-based folk singer's rousing arrangements and powerfully sincere wordplay. While many artists of the time were obsessed by creating a glamorous self-image, Chapman's stripped-down sound centred on simple melodies and affecting politically correct lyrics. Although the album was met with critical acclaim, sales of the album didn't start to soar until she played at a concert marking Nelson Mandela's 70th birthday, which was broadcast around the world. Released shortly after, the single 'Fast Car' peaking at Number Five in the UK and Number Six in the US. Subsequent singles 'Talkin' 'Bout a Revolution' and 'Baby Can I Hold You', fared less well, peaking in the US at Number 75 and Number 48 respectively.

Tracy Chapman topped the UK album chart, and managed to rise to Number Two on the *Billboard* Top 200. In February 1989, Chapman received three Grammy Awards, including Best Female Pop Vocal Performance for 'Fast Car'.

Number One singles:
None

Grammy awards: Best new artist; Best female pop vocal performance – Fast Car; Best contemporary folk recording;

Label: US & UK: Elektra

Recorded in:
California, USA

Personnel:
Tracy Chapman
Jack Holder
Ed Black
David LaFlamme
Steve Kaplan
Bob Marlette
Larry Klein
Denny Fongheiser
Paulinho Da Costa

Producer:
David Kershenbaum

1 Talkin' 'Bout A Revolution (2:38)
2 Fast Car (4:58)
3 Across The Lines (3:22)
4 Behind The Wall (1:46)
5 Baby Can I Hold You (3:16)
6 Mountains O' Things (4:37)
7 She's Got Her Ticket (3:54)
8 Why? (2:01)
9 For My Lover (3:15)
10 If Not Now (2:55)
11 For You (3:09)

Total album length: 35 minutes

TRACY CHAPMAN

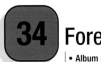

34 Forever Your Girl

| • **Album sales:** 7,300,000 | • **Release date:** June 1988 |

Having worked with some of the biggest names in 1980s pop as a highly sought-after choreographer, Paula Abdul used her industry savvy in recording her debut album *Forever Your Girl*. Not blessed with the strongest of voices, Abdul's choice of producers and her stunning videos made her a mainstay in the singles chart throughout 1989.

Forever You Girl initially languished, with the first two singles hardly making their presence known on the US charts. Despite the album's plethora of catchy pop, Abdul's breakthrough didn't come until early in 1989 when the single 'Straight Up' climbed to the peak of the *Billboard* Hot 100. Maintaining its hold for three weeks 'Straight Up' began a chain of events that would see half the songs on *Forever Your Girl* rise to the higher echelons of the singles chart.

Further Number One hits came with 'Opposites Attract', 'Cold Hearted' and the title track, while 'The Way That You Love Me' made it to Number Three. An expert in imagery, Abdul won Best Music Video, Short Form for 'Opposites Attract' at the 1990 Grammy Awards.

Number One singles:
US: Forever Your Girl;
Straight Up; Opposites
Attract; Cold Hearted

Grammy awards:
Best Music Video, Short
Form – Opposites Attract

Label: US & UK: Virgin

Recorded in:
Los Angeles, USA

Producers:
L.A. Reid
Babyface
Glen Ballard,
Jesse Johnson
Dave Cochrane

Personnel:
Paula Abdul
Oliver Leiber
Dave Cochrane
Bobby Gonzales
Basil Fung
Dann Huff
Bob Somma
Troy Williams
Eddie M
St Paul
Jesse Johnson
Kayo
Randy Weber
Ricky P
Various other personnel

1 **The Way That You Love Me** (5:22)
2 **Knocked Out** (3:52)
3 **Opposites Attract** (4:24)
4 **State Of Attraction** (4:07)
5 **I Need You** (5:01)
6 **Forever Your Girl** (4:58)
7 **Straight Up** (4:11)
8 **Next To You** (4:26)
9 **Cold Hearted** (3:51)
10 **One Or The Other** (4:10)

Total album length: 44 minutes

Paula Abdul

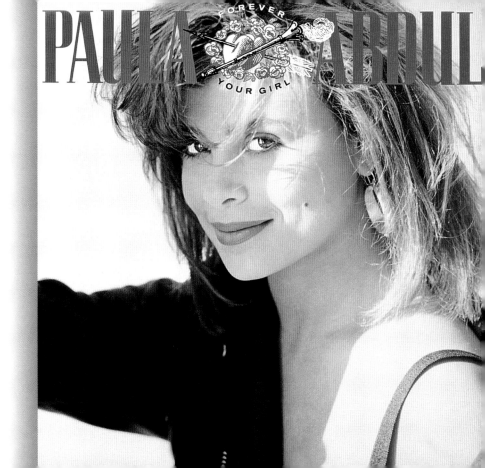

33 Don't Be Cruel

| • **Album sales:** 7,600,000 | • **Release date:** June 1988 |

Following the moderate success of his solo debut, it was Bobby Brown's sophomore album that would prove his breakthrough. Brown's use of hot new production duo L.A. Reid and Babyface and new jack pioneer Teddy Riley would prove a masterstroke. The fresh sound they provided to *Don't Be Cruel* refined the new jack swing genre and helped Brown shed his New Edition teen-pop image.

The album generated an abundance of singles, commencing with the album's title track which provided Brown with his first pop Top Ten hit. Of all the singles, 'My Prerogative' proved to be the most successful, rising to the peak of the *Billboard* Hot 100, while the upbeat dance number 'Every Little Step' and ballads 'Roni', and 'Rock Wit'cha' also made their presence known in the US Top Ten.

Meanwhile, the accompanying superbly choreographed videos played a considerable part in reshaping Brown's image while receiving heavy rotation on MTV.

Don't Be Cruel went to Number One in the *Billboard* Top 200, while the hit single 'Every Little Step' won Brown a Grammy for Best Male R&B Vocal Performance.

Number One singles:
US: My Prerogative

Grammy awards: Best male R&B performance – Every Little Step

Label: US & UK: MCA

Recorded in: N/A

Personnel:
Bobby Brown
Larry White
Emilio Conesa

Melicio Magdaluyo
Dewayne Sweet
Teddy Riley
Percy Scott
Ben Rayes
Kirk Crumpler
Flip Kirby
Various other personnel

Producers:
L.A. Reid
Babyface
Gene Griffin
Larry White
Gordon Jones

1 Cruel Prelude (0:39)
2 Don't Be Cruel (6:52)
3 My Prerogative (4:57)
4 Roni (5:58)
5 Rock Wit'cha (4:47)
6 Every Little Step (3:59)
7 I'll Be Good To You (4:25)
8 Take It Slow (5:22)
9 All Day All Night (4:40)
10 I Really Love You Girl (5:11)
11 Cruel Reprise (0:18)

Total album length: 47 minutes

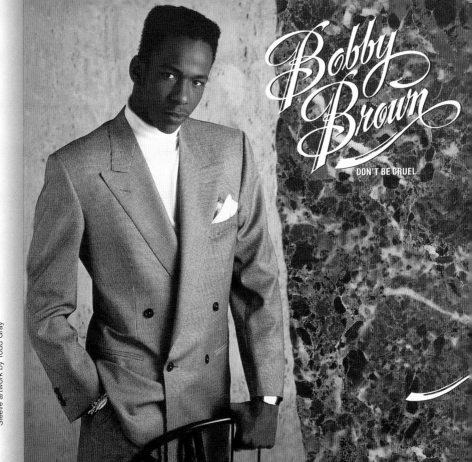

Bobby Brown

DON'T BE CRUEL

32 New Jersey

| • **Album sales:** 7,600,000 | • **Release date:** September 1988 |

Combining heavy rock with the melodious sensibilities of Bruce Springteen, Bon Jovi had rocketed to success when their previous album, *Slippery When Wet*, sold 12,000,000 copies. Celebrating the band's home state, *New Jersey* proved only slightly less popular, reaching Number One in the US, the UK, and several other countries around the world.

Like *Slippery When Wet*, the new album was produced by Bruce Fairbairn and engineered by Bob Rock at Little Mountain Sound in Vancouver. *New Jersey* found Bon Jovi honing their anthemic brand of cowboy-rock, while finding time to experiment. The track 'Ride Cowboy Ride', for example, was recorded in mono. In the end, the band recorded enough material for a double album, a plan laid to rest by their record label.

New Jersey went multi-platinum and proved a huge international success, selling seven million copies in the US alone, while generating two Number One singles, 'Bad Medicine' and 'I'll Be There for You'. Other hits included 'Born To Be My Baby', which reached Number Three, and Top Ten singles 'Lay Your Hands On Me' and 'Living In Sin'.

Number One singles:
US: Bad Medicine; I'll Be There For You

Grammy awards:
None

Label: US: Mercury;
UK: Vertigo

Recorded in:
Vancouver, Canada

Personnel:
Jon Bon Jovi
Richie Sambora
David Bryan
Alec John Such
Tico 'The Hit Man' Torres
Audrey Nordwell
Scott Fairbairn
Bruce Fairbairn
Gouin 'Dido' Morris
Audrey Nordwell
Peter Berring

Producer:
Bruce Fairbairn

1 **Lay Your Hands on Me (6:01)**
2 **Bad Medicine (5:16)**
3 **Born To Be My Baby (4:40)**
4 **Living In Sin (4:39)**
5 **Blood On Blood (6:16)**
6 **Homebound Train (5:20)**
7 **Wild Is The Wind (5:08)**
8 **Ride Cowboy Ride (1:25)**
9 **Stick To Your Guns (4:45)**
10 **I'll Be There For You (5:46)**
11 **99 In The Shade (4:28)**
12 **Love For Sale (3:58)**

Total album length: 57 minutes

Bon Jovi

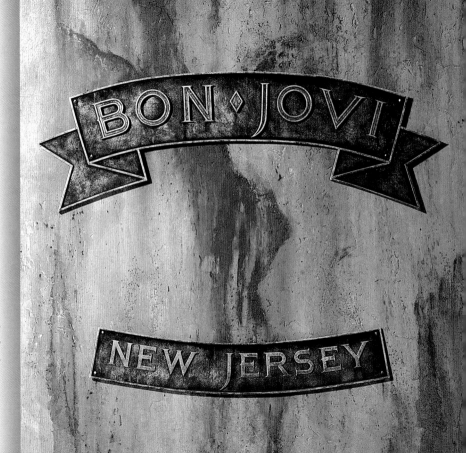

31 An Innocent Man

| • **Album sales:** 7,900,000 | • **Release date:** August 1983 |

Following the relative commercial failure of his previous album *Nylon Curtain*, Billy Joel regained his multi-platinum credentials with 1983's *An Innocent Man*. Many of the songs on the album were inspired by Joel's fiancée Christie Brinkley. Indeed, it was his romance with Brinkley that inspired 'Uptown Girl', an upbeat tribute that peaked at Number Three on the US charts and topped the UK charts. An early adopter of music videos, Joel also appeared alongside his model girlfriend in a series of clips that proved hugely popular on MTV. Other hit US singles included 'The Longest Time', 'Leave A Tender Moment Alone', 'Keeping The Faith' and the soulful single 'Tell Her About It'.

An Innocent Man is a breezy upbeat collection, a return to the music of Joel's youth. This approach provided Joel with his most successful album ever, peaking at Number Four on the *Billboard* Top 200 chart.

Number One singles:
US: Tell Her About It;
UK: Uptown Girl

Grammy awards: None

Label: US: Columbia;
UK: CBS

Recorded in:
New York, USA

Personnel:
Billy Joel
Eric Gale
Russell Javors,
David Brown
Charles McCracken
Toots Thielmans
Mark Rivera
David Sanborn
Michael Brecker
Ronnie Cuber

Joseph J. Shepley
Jon Faddis
John Gatchell
Richard Tee
Leon Pendarvis
Rob Mounsey
Doug Stegmeyer
Liberty DeVito
Ralph MacDonald
Bill Zampino
Michael Alexander
Rory Dodd
Frank Floyd
Lani Groves
Ullanda McCulloch
Ron Taylor
Terry Textor
Eric Troyer
Tom Bahler

Producers:
Phil Ramone
Billy Joel

1 **Easy Money** (4:04)
2 **An Innocent Man** (5:17)
3 **The Longest Time** (3:42)
4 **This Night** (4:17)
5 **Tell Her About It** (3:52)
6 **Uptown Girl** (3:17)
7 **Careless Talk** (3:48)
8 **Christie Lee** (3:31)
9 **Leave A Tender Moment Alone** (3:56)
10 **Keeping The Faith** (7:11)

Total album length: 40 minutes

Billy Joel

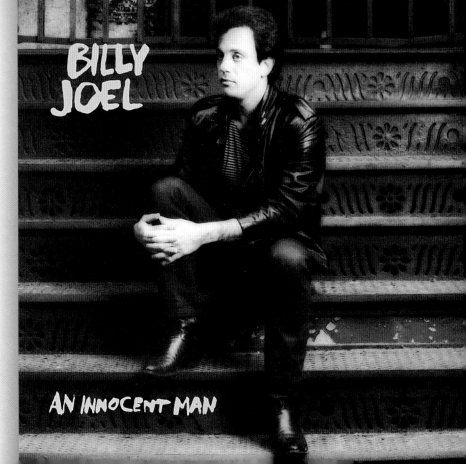

BILLY JOEL

AN INNOCENT MAN

30 Hangin' Tough

| • **Album sales:** 8,100,000 | • **Release date:** January 1988 |

New Kids On The Block were very much the brain-child of pop producer Maurice Starr. Having had huge commercial success with the act New Edition, Star attempted to replicate that achievement by recruiting five talented and attractive Boston teenagers to perform his songs.

The band's debut, *New Kids On The Block*, sold poorly when first released, but Starr's efforts paid off with their second attempt *Hangin' Tough*. The album mixed rap and pop in the same way as its predeccessor, but better material and a more streetwise image widened the band's appeal. Once again, Starr not only wrote the songs but also played almost all the instruments.

The album's first single, 'Please Don't Go Girl', reached Number Ten in the US, but it wasn't until the band joined Tiffany on tour as her opening act that sales really took off. *Hangin' Tough* produced four more Top Ten singles for the band including two US Number Ones. New Kids On the Block became a pop sensation, surrounded by screaming teenagers wherever they went and were biggest-selling band in America in 1989.

After the success of *Hangin' Tough*, the band's first album *was* re-released and peaked at Number 25. In 1994 the band, now called NKOTB, attempted to reinvent themselves as a credible R&B act. They recorded an album, *Face The Music*, without Starr but failed to recapture their success and split later that year.

Number One singles:
IUS: I'll Be Loving You (Forever); UK: You Got It (The Right Stuff); US & UK: Hangin' Tough

Grammy awards:
None

Label: US & UK: Columbia

Recorded in: N/A

Personnel:
Jordan Knight
Jon Knight
Joe McIntyre
Donnie Wahlberg
Danny Wood
Maurice Starr

Producer:
Maurice Starr

1 **You Got It (The Right Stuff) (4:09)**
2 **Please Don't Go Girl (4:30)**
3 **I'll Be Loving You (Forever) (4:22)**
4 **Cover Girl (4:02)**
5 **I Need You (3:36)**
6 **Hangin' Tough (4:16)**
7 **I Remember When (4:09)**
8 **What'cha Gonna Do About It? (3:54)**
9 **My Favourite Girl (5:28)**
10 **Hol On (3:36)**

Total album length: 42 minutes

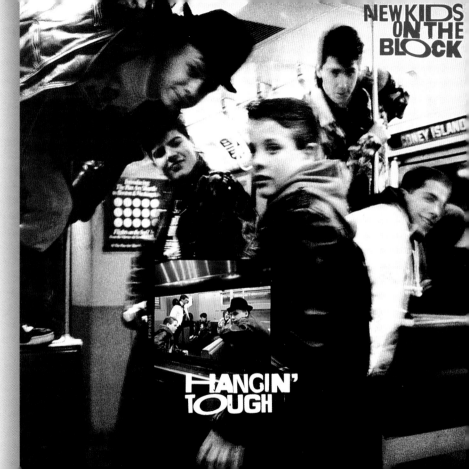

NEW KIDS
ON THE
BLOCK

CONEY ISLAND

HANGIN'
TOUGH

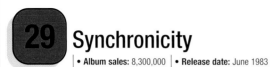

Synchronicity

| • **Album sales:** 8,300,000 | • **Release date:** June 1983 |

Synchronicity was recorded by the Police in the West Indies and Canada with the band fully aware it would be their last studio recording together. Remarkably band members seemed unaffected by the knowledge, managing to produce an outstanding album that became regarded as a benchmark from the hugely influential act. Following the album's release, the band undertook an enormous world tour before finally announcing a permanent 'sabbatical'.

The fifth Police album, Synchronicity retains a loose theme based on C.G. Jung's psychosocial connecting principle. The album generated a string of hit singles including 'King of Pain', 'Wrapped Around Your Finger' and the ballad 'Every Breath You Take' which was written by Sting in a ten-minute burst of inspiration in the middle of the night.

Synchronicity spent two weeks in top position on the UK chart; its 17-week run as a US Number One album was even more impressive. The single 'Every Breath You Take' went to Number One in the UK and spent eight weeks at the peak of the US chart, becoming one of the country's biggest-selling singles.

Number One singles:
US & UK: Every Breath You Take

Grammy awards: Best pop performance by a duo or group; Best rock performance by a duo or group

Label: US & UK: A&M

Recorded in: Montserrat, West Indies & Quebec, Canada

Personnel:
Andy Summers
Sting
Stewart Copeland

Producers:
Hugh Padgham
Andy Summers
Sting
Stewart Copeland

1 **Synchronicity I** (3:23)
2 **Walking In Your Footsteps** (3:36)
3 **O My God** (4:02)
4 **Mother** (3:05)
5 **Miss Gradenko** (1:59)
6 **Synchronicity II** (5:02)
7 **Every Breath You Take** (4:13)
8 **King Of Pain** (4:59)
9 **Wrapped Around Your Finger** (5:13)
10 **Tea In The Sahara** (4:19)
11 **Murder By Numbers** (4:36)

Total album length: 44 minutes

The Police

THE POLICE

SYNCHRONICITY

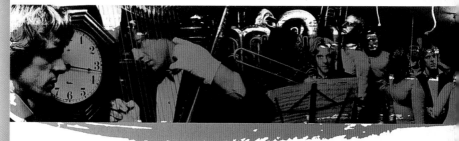

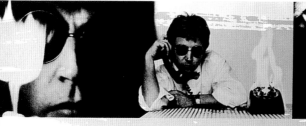

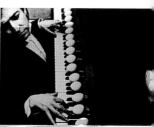

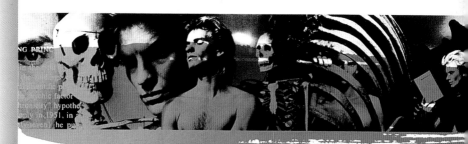

28 Eliminator

| • Album sales: 8,900,000 | • Release date: March 1983 |

ZZ Top's tongue-in-cheek machismo, endearing image and experimental form of catchy, riff-laden rock came together perfectly on *Eliminator*. Released in 1983 the album broke new ground for the band. Although it never managed to attain a position higher than Number Nine on the US album chart, it kept a foothold in the Top 20 for over a year. The reception in the UK was no less spectacular, as *Eliminator* peaked at Number Three.

Like many of the most successful 1980s acts, ZZ Top were quick to realize the power of the new MTV network. The videos produced in support of the album were firmly tongue-in-cheek, relying on the the Texan trio's instantly recognisable beard 'n' shades image. Oddly, the middle-aged men, who had been together since 1970, became both hip and endearing, leading to considerable television airplay. On one memorable occasion, the band appeared on *The Tonight Show* with a bearded Johnny Carson.

Eliminator spawned a string of memorable singles, including 'Gimme All Your Lovin',' 'Sharp Dressed Man' and 'Legs', the latter peaking at Number Eight on the *Billboard* Hot 100.

Another contributing factor to the album's commercial success was the polished production of Bill Ham. The producer expanded greatly the role of synthesizers, in evidence on the previous *Deguello* and *El Loco* albums, adding sheen to the trio's hard blues sound.

Number One singles:
None

Grammy awards: None

Label: US & UK: Warner

Recorded in:
Memphis, Tennessee

Personnel:
Billy Gibbons
Dusty Hill
Frank Beard

Producers:
Bill Ham

1 Gimme All Your Lovin' (3:59)
2 Got Me Under Pressure (3:59)
3 Sharp Dressed Man (4:13)
4 I Need You Tonight (6:14)
5 I Got The Six (2:52)
6 Legs (4:35)
7 Thug (4:17)
8 TV Dinners (3:50)
9 Dirty Dog (4:05)
10 If I Could Only Flag Her Down (3:40)
11 Bad Girl (3:16)

Total album length: 45 minutes

ZZ Top

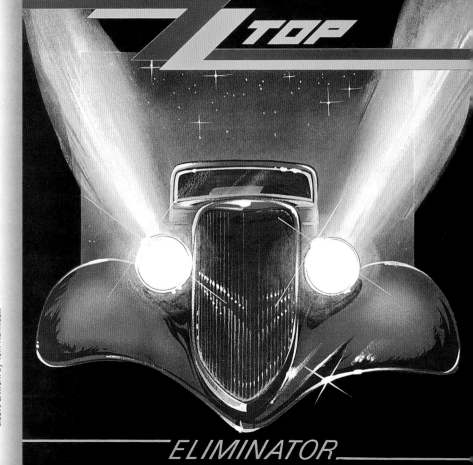

sleeve artwork by Tom Hunnicutt

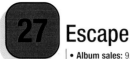

27 Escape

• Album sales: 9,000,000 | **• Release date:** August 1981

Journey's bid for commercial acceptance began in 1978 with the addition of 18-year-old vocalist Steve Perry to the line-up and was crystallized with the release of *Escape* in 1981. Two additional line-up changes also contributed to that album's success. In 1979, Drummer Aynsley Dunbar left the band. He was replaced by Steve Smith, formerly of Montrose, who already had experience of touring with the group – Smith would go on to contribute heavily towards the compositions on *Escape*.

Two years later, keyboard player Gregg Rolie also departed, and at his suggestion, was replaced by Jonathan Cain of the Babys. Cain's versatility as a guitarist, keyboard player and singer allowed the group a new level of flexibility.

With the new line-up in place, Journey released a hugely successful double live album, *Captured*, which reached Number Nine on the US charts. The success of *Captured*, combined with the popularity of 'Open Arms', which had appeared on the *Heavy Metal* soundtrack, paved the way for the commercial success of *Escape*.

In an attempt to capture the spark of their live performances, Journey hired Kevin Elson to produce *Escape*. Elson had previously worked on tour with the group as a sound engineer.

The album's success was due in large part to the three strong singles 'Who's Crying Now', 'Don't Stop Believin'' and 'Open Arms', each of which also made it to the US Top Ten.

Number One singles:
None

Grammy awards: None

Label: US: Columbia;
UK: CBS

Recorded in:
Berkeley, California.

Personnel:
Steve Perry
Jonathan Cain
Neil Schon
Ross Valory
Steve Smith

Producer:
Kevin Elson

1 Don't Stop Believin' (4:10)
2 Stone In Love (4:25)
3 Who's Crying Now (5:01)
4 Keep On Runnin' (3:39)
5 Still They Ride (3:49)
6 Escape (5:16)
7 Lay It Down (4:13)
8 Dead Or Alive (3:20)
9 Mother, Father (5:28)
10 Open Arms (3:18)

Total album length: 43 minutes

Journey

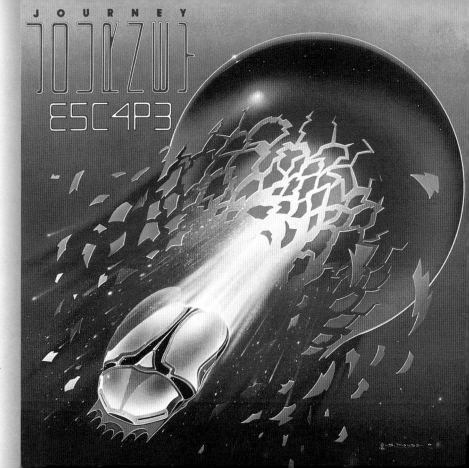

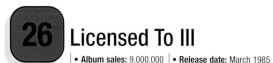

26 Licensed To Ill

| • **Album sales:** 9,000,000 | • **Release date:** March 1985 |

Following high-profile concert tours with Madonna and Run-DMC, Brooklyn's Beastie Boys made history with their much anticipated full-length debut, *License To Ill*. Mixing rap with heavy rock riffs, the innovative and thoroughly irreverent album went platinum within two months of its release and became the first rap album to reach Number One on the *Billboard* Top 200 chart. The reception on the other side of the Atlantic was also impressive. The album reached Number Seven in the UK.

The hugely original feel of the album was largely due to the work of producer-DJ Rick Rubin who sampled infectious licks from the likes Led Zeppelin and James Brown to create mammoth hooks for the act's raps to hang on, while exposing a sizeable sense of humour. With its tongue-in-cheek obnoxiousness, the Beastie Boys' debut proved hugely popular and not a little controversial. Fraternity brat anthem '(You Gotta) Fight for Your Right (To Party!)' may well have reached Number Seven on the *Billboard* Hot 100, but their flippancy caused the act to be regarded as pariahs by the rap community; meanwhile, mischievously sexists tracks such as 'Girls' prompted further outcry. Combining hip-hop, and rock with mixing innovation and punk attitude *Licensed To Ill* was wholly original and helped rap become universally popular.

Number One singles:	**Personnel:**
None	Adam 'Ad-Rock' Horovitz
	Adam 'MCA' Yauch
Grammy awards:	Mike 'Mike D' Diamond
None	Kerry King
Label: US & UK: Def Jam	**Producers:**
	Rick Rubin
Recorded in:	Adam 'Ad-Rock' Horovitz
New York, USA	Adam 'MCA' Yauch
	Mike 'Mike D' Diamond

1 **Rhymin & Stealin** (4:08)
2 **The New Style** (4:36)
3 **She's Crafty** (3:35)
4 **Posse In Effect** (2:27)
5 **Slow Ride** (2:56)
6 **Girls** (3:14)
7 **Fight For Your Right** (3:28)
8 **No Sleep Till Brooklyn** (4:07)
9 **Paul Revere** (3:41)
10 **Hold It Now, Hit It** (3:26)
11 **Brass Monkey** (2:37)
12 **Slow And Low** (3:38)
13 **Time To Get Ill** (3:37)

Total album length: 45 minutes

Beastie Boys

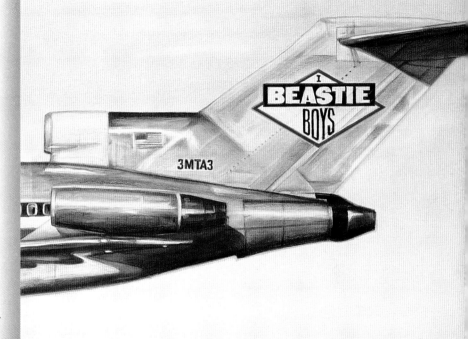

25 Garth Brooks

| • Album sales: 9,000,000 | • Release date: April 1989 |

Having made a modest living as a bar singer, Garth Brooks' eponymous debut album would be his first of many multi-platinum sellers thrusting him into the limelight and onto a remarkable career path on which he would become one of the biggest earners in the American country scene. Released in 1989, *Garth Brooks* was recorded in Nashville and produced by Allen Reynolds who had previously worked with Don Williams. A blending of traditional country with rock 'n' roll, it became the best-selling country album of the 1980s.

One of the album's strongest tracks, the romantic 'If Tomorrow Never Knows,' provided Brooks with his first Number One on the *Billboard* Hot Country chart, a feat repeated with 'The Dance'. Two other singles, 'Not Counting You' and 'Much Too Young', also made the Country Top Ten. *Garth Brooks* peaked at Number 13 on the *Billboard* Top 200 chart, and reached Number Two on the Country chart.

Number One singles:
None

Grammy awards:
None

Label: US & UK: Capitol

Recorded in:
Nashville, USA

Personnel:
Garth Brooks
Mark Casstevens
Chris Leuzinger
Bruce Bouton
Rob Hajacos
Bobby Wood
Mike Chapman
Milton Sledge
Wayland Patton
Kathy Chiavola
Hurshel Wiginton
Jennifer O'Brien
Wendy Johnson
Curtis Young
Trisha Yearwood
Carl Gorodetzky
Dennis Molchan
Pamela Sixfin
George Binkly III
Roy Christensen
Gary Vanosdale

Producer:
Allen Reynold

1 Not Counting You (2:34)
2 I've Got A Good Thing Going (2:54)
3 If Tomorrow Never Comes (3:40)
4 Uptown Down Home Good Ol' Boy (2:34)
5 Everytime That It Rains (4:12)
6 Alabama Clay (3:40)
7 Much Too Young (To Feel This Damn Old) (2:58)
8 Cowboy Bill (4:34)
9 Nobody Gets Off In This Town (2:19)
10 I Know One (2:55)
11 The Dance (3:42)

Total album length: 32 minutes

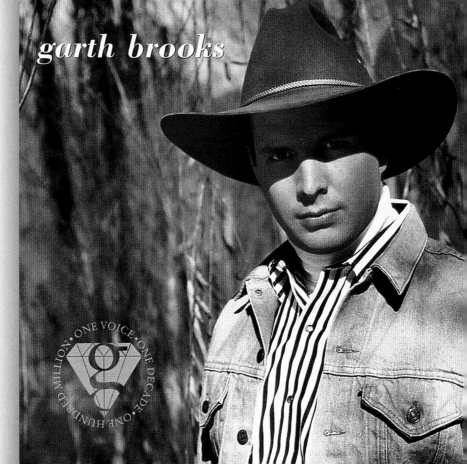

garth brooks

ONE VOICE • ONE DECADE • ONE HUNDRED MILLION

Hi Infidelity

| • **Album sales:** 9,100,000 | • **Release date:** December 1980 |

Having been regulars on the live circuit for ten years, REO Speedwagon finally hit it big with their ninth studio album in late 1980. *Hi Infidelity*, is a quintessentially 1980s album, bulging with romantic, if bombastic, ballads.

Starting out on tour as an opening act in support of the album, the band soon found their fortunes had changed. The summer of 1981 saw them headlining in arenas throughout North America. The album catapulted the band to multi-platinum status, topped the US chart, and reached Number Five in the UK.

Hi Infidelity was recorded in a week long session at the Crystal recording studio in Hollywood. During this period lead vocalist Kevin Cronin took 'Don't Let Me Down', a song written by guitarist Gary Richrath, and honed its sound and renamed it. The result was 'Take It On The Run', a bitter ballad which would go to Number Five in the US chart and manage to reach Number 17 in the UK.

However, much of the album's commercial success rests with the first single, 'Keep On Loving You', which went to Number One in the US singles chart, and gave the band its only UK Top Ten hit by peaking at Number Seven.

Number One singles:
US: Keep on Lovin' You

Grammy awards:
None

Label: US & UK: Epic

Recorded in:
Hollywood, USA

Personnel:
Kevin Cronin
Neal Doughty
Steve Foreman

Alan Gratzer
Bruce Hall
Tom Kelly
Richard Page
Gary Richrath
N. Yolletta

Producers:
Kevin Cronin
Alan Gratzer
Gary Richrath
Kevin Beamish

1 **Don't Let Him Go (3:46)**
2 **Keep On Loving You (3:22)**
3 **Follow My Heart (3:50)**
4 **In Your Letter (3:17)**
5 **Take It On The Run (4:01)**
6 **Tough Guys (3:50)**
7 **Out Of Season (3:07)**
8 **Shakin' It Loose (2:25)**
9 **Someone Tonight (2:40)**
10 **I Wish You Were There (4:27)**

Total album length: 34 minutes

REO Speedwagon

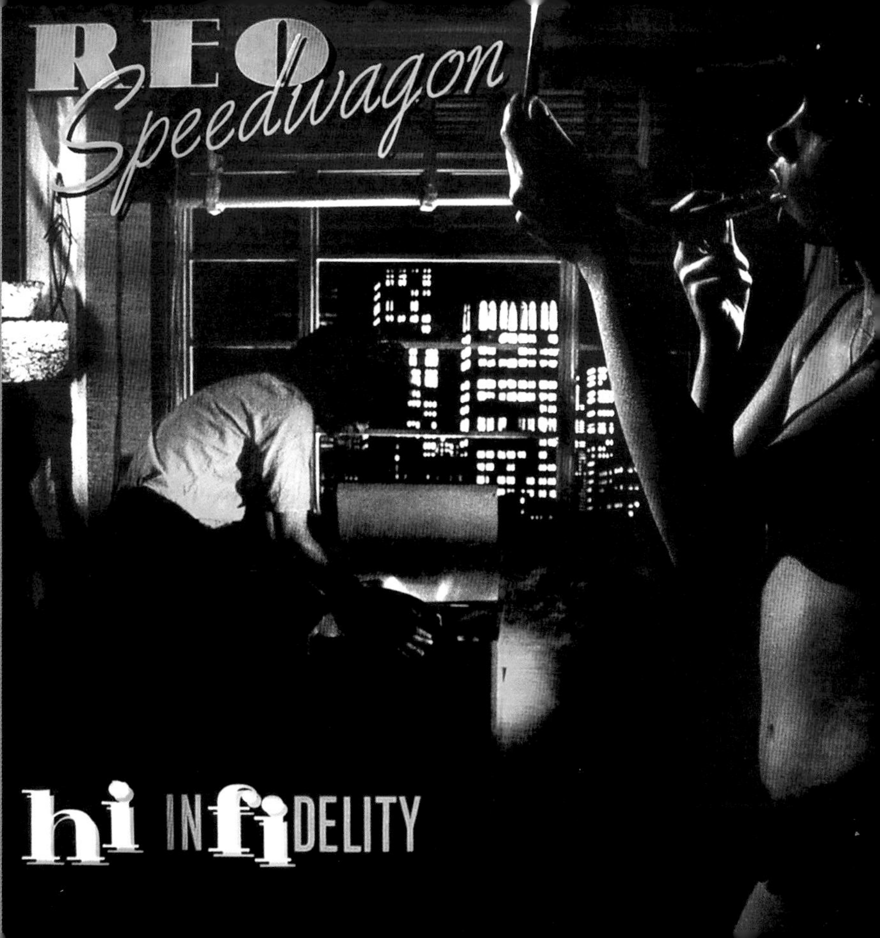
REO Speedwagon
hi INfiDELITY

23 Pyromania

| • **Album sales:** 9,100,000 | • **Release date:** February 1983 |

Def Leppard had already developed a healthy reputation before *Pyromania* brought them worldwide success. The recording of the album had been temporarily jeopardized when guitarist Pete Willis was fired and replaced with Phil Collen, formerly of glam rock group Girl.

Producer 'Mutt' Lange was retained from the previous album and continued to clean up the group's sound, placing a high emphasis on melody, smoothing out drums and guitars to perfection, and recording multi-layered vocal harmonies. Another factor, as was so often the case during the 1980s, was MTV. Def Leppard were good looking enough to draw attention on their own merits, but well-conceived videos for 'Photograph' and 'Rock of Ages' resulted in strong exposure on the young network. Not surprisingly the British band's fan base shifted from the UK to the US.

While *Pyromania* peaked at Number 16 in the UK, the album fared better across the Atlantic, where it reached the Number Two spot and stayed on the *Billboard* chart for 92 weeks.

Both 'Photograph' and 'Rock Of Ages' became US Top 20 singles (reaching Number 12 and Number 16, respectively), but failed to crack the Top 40 in the UK.

Number One singles:
None

Grammy awards:
None

Label: US: Mercury;
UK: Vertigo

Recorded in: Sussex
and London, UK

Personnel:
Joe Elliot
Steve Clark
Phil Collen
Pete Willis
Rick Savage
Rick Allen
John Kongos
Booker T. Boffin

Producer:
Robert John 'Mutt' Lange
John Kongos

1 Rock Rock ('Til You Drop) (3:52)
2 Photograph (4:12)
3 Stagefright (3:46)
4 Too Late For Love (4:30)
5 Die Hard The Hunter (6:17)
6 Foolin' (4:32)
7 Rock Of Ages (4:09)
8 Comin' Under Fire (4:20)
9 Action! Not Words (3:52)
10 Billy's Got A Gun (5:27)

Total album length: 45 minutes

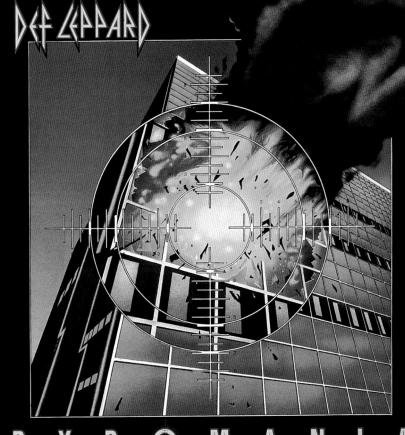

22 Footloose

| • Album sales: 9,100,000 | • Release date: March 1984 |

The *Footloose* soundtrack initially comes across as a precursor to the run of slick packages that would prove a major selling force for films of the 1980s. However, for *Footloose* in particular the music had to provide a major plot element, not just a few catchy background tracks. With this in mind all the songs used on the soundtrack were actually composed after the film had been completed in order to tie in as closely as possible with certain key scenes. For even greater cohesion, every track was co-written by screenwriter Dean Pitchford, working alongside some of the top talent of the day, including Kenny Loggins, Jim Steinman, Sammy Hagar and Ann Wilson from Heart. Another big name was Eric Carmen, who was invited to write a love theme. Carmen met with Pitchford for breakfast one morning, and completed 'Almost Paradise' before the day was out.

The soundtrack topped the US chart and was subsequently nominated for a Grammy (with Pitchford sharing the nomination with Kenny Loggins, Eric Carmen, Tom Snow, Jim Steinman, Sammy Hagar, Tom Snow, and Micheal Gore). Two songs, 'Footloose' and 'Let's Hear It For The Boy', were also nominated for Best Song at the 1985 Academy Awards.

Number One singles:
US: Footloose

Grammy awards:
None

Label: US & UK: Columbia

Recorded in:
Los Angeles, USA

Personnel:
Kenny Loggins
Deniece Williams
Ann Wilson
Mike Reno
Bonnie Tyler
Ian Lloyd
Bill Church
Karla Bonoff
Sammy Hagar
Keith Olsen
Various other personnel

Producers:
Mick Jones
David Foster
Robert John 'Mutt' Lange
Jim Steinman
Various other producers

1 Footloose (Kenny Loggins) (3:47)
2 Let's Hear It For The Boy (Deniece Williams) (4:22)
3 Almost Paradise (Love Theme from *Footloose*) (Ann Wilson & Mike Reno) (3:49)
4 Holding Out For A Hero (Bonnie Tyler) (5:50)
5 Dancing (Shalamar) (4:05)
6 I'm Free (Heaven Helps the Man) (Kenny Loggins) (3:46)
7 Somebody's Eyes (Karla Bonoff) (3:27)
8 The Girl Gets Around (Sammy Hagar) (3:23)
9 Never (Moving Picture) (3:47)

Total album length: 36 minutes

Original Soundtrack

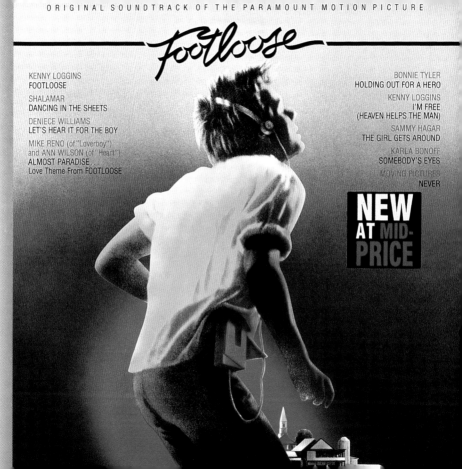

ORIGINAL SOUNDTRACK OF THE PARAMOUNT MOTION PICTURE

Footloose

KENNY LOGGINS
FOOTLOOSE

SHALAMAR
DANCING IN THE SHEETS

DENIECE WILLIAMS
LET'S HEAR IT FOR THE BOY

MIKE RENO (of "Loverboy")
and ANN WILSON (of "Heart")
ALMOST PARADISE...
Love Theme From FOOTLOOSE

BONNIE TYLER
HOLDING OUT FOR A HERO

KENNY LOGGINS
I'M FREE
(HEAVEN HELPS THE MAN)

SAMMY HAGAR
THE GIRL GETS AROUND

KARLA BONOFF
SOMEBODY'S EYES

MOVING PICTURES
NEVER

NEW
AT MID-
PRICE

21 True Blue

| • **Album sales:** 9,100,000 | • **Release date:** June 1986 |

Having established her pop music credentials with the Number One album *Like A Virgin*, Madonna set out to secure critical recognition with her third album *True Blue*. Despite admitting to knowing little, at that time, about the technical side of recording, Madonna opted to co-produce the album alongside Patrick Leonard and Stephen Bray. The resulting sound was cleaner and simpler than the lush pop production on *Like A Virgin*, emphasising songwriting over effect.

Although some of the songs were composed while on tour, Madonna started writing in earnest for *True Blue* prior to filming *Shanghai Surprise* with then-husband Sean Penn. The title track was written as a love song to Penn, while 'Live To Tell' was to become the theme-song to his movie *At Close Range*.

'Live To Tell,' the first single, was released a month before the album and went to Number One in the US. She repeated the acheivement with two subsequent singles, the controversial 'Papa Don't Preach' and 'Open Your Heart'. The two other singles, 'True Blue' and 'La Isla Bonita' were also Top Five hits in her native land.

Number One singles:
US & UK: Papa Don't Preach; US: Live To Tell; Open Your Heart; UK: True Blue; La Isla Bonita

Grammy awards: None

Label: US & UK: Sire

Recorded in:
Various locations

Producers:
Madonna
Stephen Bray
Patrick Leonard

Personnel:
Madonna
Richard Marx
David Williams
Johnathan Moffett
Dann Huff
Paul Jackson Jr
Bruce Gaitsch
John Putnam
Dave Boroff
Stephen Bray
Pat Leonard
Fred Zarr
Paulinho Da Costa
Kiethan Carter
Jackie Jackson
Various other personnel

1   Papa Don't Preach (4.29)
2   Open Your Heart (4.13)
3   White Heat (4.40)
4   Live To Tell (5.52)
5   Where's The Party (4.21)
6   True Blue (4.18)
7   La Isla Bonita (4.02)
8   Jimmy, Jimmy (3.55)
9   Love Makes The World Go Round (4.35)

Total album length: 40 minutes

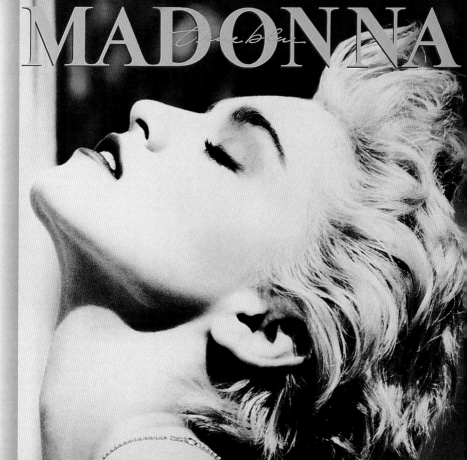

MADONNA

20 Top Gun

| • Album sales: 9,600,000 | • Release date: May 1986 |

One of the best-selling soundtracks of all time, *Top Gun* remains a quintessential collection of 1980s pop. The film, meanwhile, made a star of the young Tom Cruise, while boosting the careers of Tim Robbins and Meg Ryan.

Two singles dominate the album, Berlin's massive hit, 'Take My Breath Away', which acts as the centrepiece and Kenny Loggins' 'Danger Zone', both co-written by Italian electronica specialist Giorgio Moroder, who previously scored *Midnight Express*. Canada's Loverboy provided a third single, 'Heaven In Your Eyes', which reached Number 12 on the US chart.

The soundtrack went to Number One in the US while Berlin's 'Take My Breath Away' hit Number One in the US and UK, where it stayed for 15 weeks to become the ninth best-selling single in British chart history. The track also won an Oscar for Best Song. Further critical acclaim followed at the Grammys, where Harold Faltermeyer and Steve Stevens won the award for Best Pop Instrumental Performance for 'Top Gun Anthem'.

Number One singles:
US & UK: Take My Breath Away

Grammy awards:
Best pop instrumental performance – Top Gun Anthem

Label: US & UK: Columbia

Recorded in:
Various locations

Personnel:
Kenny Loggins
Cheap Trick
Terri Nunn
Ric Olsen
Gloria Estefan
Mike Reno
Matthew Frenette
Scott Smith
Larry Greene
Marietta
Harold Faltermeyer
Steve Stevens
Various other personnel

Producers:
Peter Wolf
Paul Dean
Phil Spector
Giorgio Moroder
Sam Phillips
Various other producers

1 Danger Zone (Kenny Loggins) (3:36)
2 Mighty Wings (Cheap Trick) (3:51)
3 Playing With the Boys (Kenny Loggins) (3:59)
4 Lead Me On (Teena Marie) (3:47)
5 Take My Breath Away (Love Theme from *Top Gun*) (Berlin) (4:15)
6 Hot Summer Nights (Miami Sound Machine) (3:38)
7 Heaven in Your Eyes (Loverboy) (4:04)
8 Through the Fire (Larry Greene) (3:45)
9 Destination Unknown (Marietta) (3:48)
10 Top Gun Anthem (Harold Faltermeyer & Steve Stevens) (4:13)

Total album length: 37 minutes

Original Soundtrack

TOP GUN

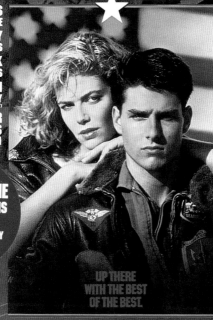

KENNY LOGGINS
DANGER ZONE

LOVERBOY
HEAVEN IN YOUR EYES

CHEAP TRICK
MIGHTY WINGS

BERLIN
TAKE MY BREATH AWAY
(LOVE THEME FROM "TOP GUN")

**HAROLD FALTERMEYER
& STEVE STEVENS**
TOP GUN ANTHEM

Includes the single
DANGER ZONE
by **KENNY LOGGINS**

plus the U.S. No. 1

TAKE MY BREATH AWAY
by **BERLIN**

CBS 70296

**MIAMI SOUND
MACHINE**
HOT SUMMER NIGHTS

KENNY LOGGINS
PLAYING WITH THE BOYS

TEENA MARIE
LEAD ME ON

MARIETTA
DESTINATION UNKNOWN

LARRY GREENE
THROUGH THE FIRE

UP THERE
WITH THE BEST
OF THE BEST.

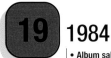

19 1984

• Album sales: 10,100,000 | **• Release date:** January 1984

Frustrated by his experiences while recording the band's two previous albums, Eddie Van Halen made stringent efforts to exercise greater artistic control with *1984*. A major step included setting up his own studio, where he insisted the album be recorded. He was also successful in persuading his fellow members to allow the use of synthesizers in their music.

Van Halen already had several platinum albums to its name, but Eddie Van Halen was keen to move away from the play-it-safe attitude of the past. Ironically, with *1984* the group would achieve bigger sales than ever before. This was in part due to Eddie Van Halen's performance on Michael Jackson's 'Beat It', which had been a massive hit the previous year. Perhaps learning

from Jackson's example, Van Halen also set about filming entertaining videos for the various single releases, which helped add a TV-based audience to their fanbase.

Released only nine days into the year for which it was named, the album achieved Number Two position in the US and Number 15 in the UK.

Eddie Van Halen's enthusiasm for synthesizers was vindicated when 'Jump' became a massive hit, reaching Number One in the US and Number Four in the UK. 'Panama' and 'I'll Wait' provided two more US Top 20 hits.

The album reached multi-platinum status well before the end of the year, but the success exacerbated existing tensions within the band, and singer Dave Lee Roth quit the following year.

Number One singles:
US: Jump

Grammy awards: None

Label: US & UK: Warner

Recorded in:
California, USA

Personnel:
David Lee Roth
Eddie Van Halen
Michael Anthony
Alex Van Halen

Producer:
Ted Templeman

1 1984 (1:07)
2 Jump (4:04)
3 Panama (3:32)
4 Top Jimmy (3:02)
5 Drop Dead Legs (4:15)
6 Hot For Teacher (4:44)
7 I'll Wait (4:45)
8 Girl Gone Bad (4:35)
9 House Of Pain (3:19)

Total album length: 33 minutes

Van Halen

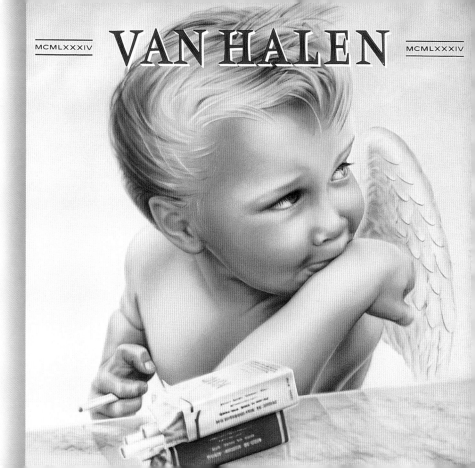

18 Whitney

| • **Album sales:** 10,800,000 | • **Release date:** May 1987 |

Whitney Houston had enjoyed three consecutive Number One hits with tracks from her debut album. She continued the run with songs from her second album, *Whitney*, which sent her into the record books as the first artist ever to have seven consecutive Number Ones in the US. No stranger to breaking records, Houston had earlier made history when *Whitney* became the first album by a female artist to debut at Number One in the *Billboard* chart.

The core production team from her first album, Narada Michael Walden, Michael Masser and Kashif, all returned, ensuring that Houston's crossover appeal was maintained. Sure enough, the first single, 'I Wanna Dance With Somebody', topped several different *Billboard* charts, including Adult Contemporary, R&B, and the Hot 100 (not to mention the UK singles chart).

By this time Whitney was confident enough to record her own rendering of the show tune 'I Know Him So Well', duetting with her own mother, Cissy Houston.

Although *Whitney* contained no less than four US number one hits, sales fell a few million short of Houston's debut album.

Number One singles:
US & UK: I Wanna Dance with Somebody (Who Loves Me); US: Didn't We Almost Have It All; So Emotional; Where Do Broken Hearts Go

Grammy awards:
Best female pop vocal performance

Label: US & UK: Arista

Recorded in: N/A

Personnel:
Whitney Houston
Cissy Houston
Paul Jackson Jr
Kenny G
Kashif
Robbie Buchanan
Randy Jackson
Roy Ayers
Paulinho Da Costa
Various other personnel

Producers:
John 'Jellybean' Benitez
Narada Michael Walden
Michael Masser
Kashif

1 I Wanna Dance With Somebody (Who Loves Me) (4:52)
2 Just The Lonely Talking Again (5:34)
3 Love Will Save The Day (5:25)
4 Didn't We Almost Have It All (5:07)
5 So Emotional (4:37)
6 Where You Are (4:11)
7 Love Is A Contact Sport (4:19)
8 You're Still My Man (4:18)
9 For The Love Of You (5:33)
10 Where Do Broken Hearts Go (4:38)
11 I Know Him So Well (4:30)

Total album length: 53 minutes

Whitney

17 Can't Slow Down

• **Album sales:** 10,900,000 • **Release date:** October 1983

Lionel Richie's rise to solo superstardom parallels with that of his 'We Are The World' co-writer Michael Jackson. Both had become the main attraction in the groups they performed with, and had achieved enviable success with their first solo albums. Richie had already given Motown its biggest single to date ('Endless Love', performed with Diana Ross). However, as with Jackson, these early triumphs were eclipsed by the release of his second solo album, *Can't Slow Down*, in 1983.

During his Commodores career, Richie had gradually steered the band away from rigid soul and funk towards a more commercial pop sound. This shift was fully realised with *Can't Slow Down*, Motown's biggest selling album. It won Richie Grammys for Album of the Year and Producer of the Year, an honour he shared with David Foster and James Anthony Carmichael.

Five of the album's tracks, 'All Night Long', 'Penny Lover', 'Stuck on You', 'Running with the Night' and 'Hello' went on to become hit singles in the US. In 1984, Richie performed 'All Night Long' before a worldwide audience at the closing ceremony of the Los Angeles Olympics.

Number One singles:
US & UK: Hello

Grammy awards: Album of the year; Producer of the year (non-classical)

Label: US & UK: Motown

Recorded in:
California, USA

Personnel:
Lionel Richie
David Cochrane
Sonny Burke
Darrell Jones
Carlos Rios
Steve Lukather
Louie Shelton
John Hobbs
Reginald 'Sonny' Burke
David Foster
Michael Boddicker
Greg Phillinganes
Abraham Laboriel
Nathan East
Paul Leim
John Robinson
Jeff Porcaro
Paulinho Da Costa
Richard Marx
Malinda Chatman
Various other personnel

Producers:
Lionel Richie
James Anthony Carmichael
David Foster

1   Can't Slow Down (4:43)
2   All Night Long (All Night) (6:25)
3   Penny Lover (5:35)
4   Stuck On You (3:15)
5   Love Will Find A Way (6:16)
6   The Only One (4:24)
7   Running With The Night (6:02)
8   Hello (4:11)

Total album length: 41 minutes

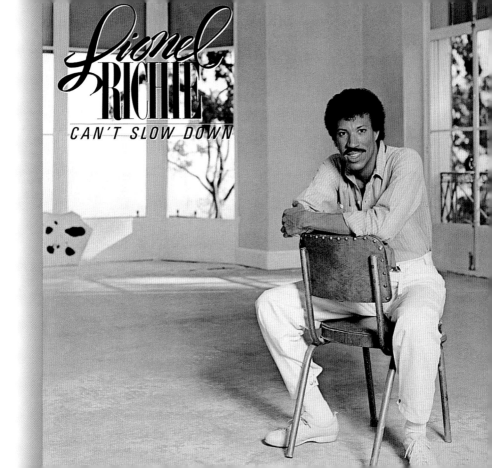

16 Like A Virgin

| • **Album sales:** 10,900,000 | • **Release date:** November 1984 |

Madonna had already reached the top ten with singles from her first album. However, it was the release of *Like A Virgin* that not only turned her into a superstar, but saw her become one of the lasting cultural icons of the 1980s.

Always far more astute than her early image might have suggested, Madonna carefully planned her next assault on the world. She brought in former Chic guitarist Nile Rodgers, the producer of David Bowie's recent *Let's Dance*, to produce the album. *Like A Virgin* was completed sometime before the buzz around Madonna's first self-titled album began to die down. In fact,

the release of 'Like A Virgin', the first single from the album, had to be delayed while the Top Five single 'Lucky Star', from *Madonna*, gradually climbed down the charts.

When released, 'Like A Virgin' topped the charts in the US and reached Number Three in the UK. At its peak, the single was selling 75,000 copies per day in the US alone. Three other singles followed: 'Material Girl', 'Angel' and 'Dress You Up', all of which became Top Five hits on both sides of the Atlantic.

Like A Virgin was certified platinum the month after release, and was six times platinum by the end of the following year.

Number One singles:
US: Like A Virgin

Grammy awards:
None

Label: US & UK: Sire

Recorded in:
New York, USA

Producer:
Nile Rogers

Personnel:
Madonna
Nile Rodgers
Lenny Pickett
Rob Sabino
Bernard Edwards
Tony Thompson
Jimmy Bralower
Curtis King,
Frank Simms,
George Simms,
Brenda King

1 **Material Girl** (4:01)
2 **Angel** (3:55)
3 **Like A Virgin** (3:39)
4 **Over And Over** (4:12)
5 **Love Don't Live Here Anymore** (4:50)
6 **Dress You Up** (4:01)
7 **Shoo-Bee-Doo** (5:17)
8 **Pretender** (4:30)
9 **Stay** (4:06)

Total album length: 38 minutes

Madonna

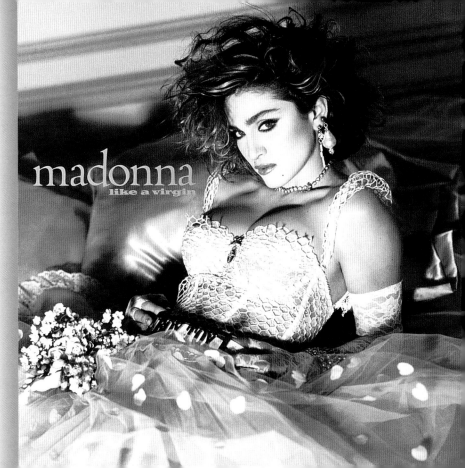

madonna
like a virgin

15 Faith

| • **Album sales:** 11,200,000 | • **Release date:** October 1987 |

Following a brief period away from the public eye, with only the release of the single 'A Different Corner' to otherwise help shed his Wham! image, George Michael commenced his bid for solo stardom in 1988 with the release of 'I Want Your Sex'. Complete with a controversial video, the single was promptly banned by a number of radio stations and thereby secured Michael the publicity to ensure that his debut solo album, *Faith*, was a massive success.

Clearly conscious of the need to prove himself as a serious musician in both the public and the critical eye, George Michael not only wrote all the songs on *Faith*, but also produced, and arranged the album, performed most of the vocal tracks, played many of the instruments, and even had a hand in the sleeve design.

Faith went to Number One in both the UK and the US, with George Michael becoming the first white solo artist to top the *Billboard* R&B album chart. The album was particularly well-received in the US, producing four Number One singles and earning a Grammy Award. Peaking at Number Two, 'Faith' was the most successful of the singles on the UK chart.

Number One singles:
US: Faith; Father Figure; Monkey; One More Try

Grammy awards:
Album of the year

Label: US: Columbia; UK: Epic

Recorded in: Denmark & London, UK

Personnel:
George Michael
Hugh Burns
Lord Monty

Lee Fothergill
J.J. Belle
Roddy Matthews
Robert Ahwai
John Altman
Mark Chandler
Steve Waterman
Malcolm Griffiths
Jamie Talbot
Steve Sidwell
Paul Spong
Shirley Lewis
Various other personnel

Producers:
George Michael
David Austin

1 Faith (3:16)
2 Father Figure (5:36)
3 I Want Your Sex, Pt. 1 & 2 (9:17)
4 One More Try (5:50)
5 Hard Day (4:48)
6 Hand To Mouth (4:36
7 Look At Your Hands (4:37)
8 Monkey (5:05)
9 Kissing A Fool (4:35)
10 Hard Day (Remix) (6:30)
11 A Last Request (I Want Your Sex, Pt. 3) (3:48)

Total album length: 53 minutes

George Michael

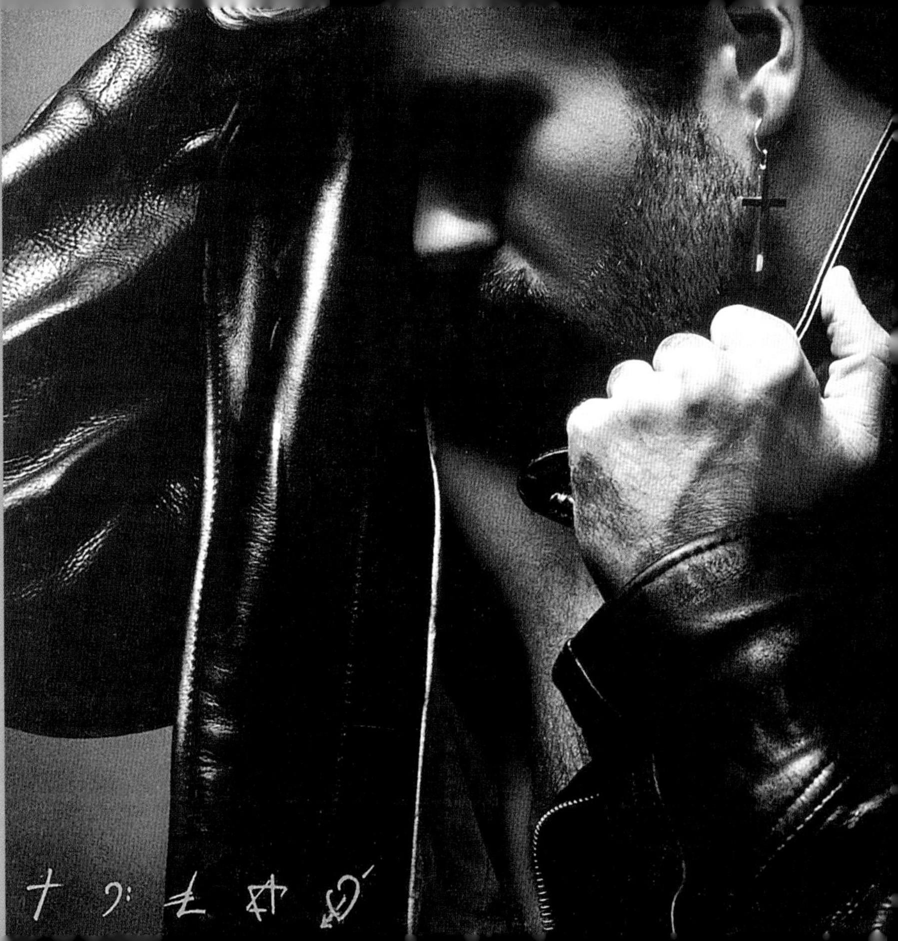

The Joshua Tree

| • **Album sales:** 11,800,000 | • **Release date:** March 1987 |

Even before 1987, U2 were well on their way to becoming one of the world's biggest bands, with a performance on Live Aid in 1985 bringing them worldwide attention. The release of *The Joshua Tree* two years later was eagerly anticipated and the album set a new record by going platinum within 28 hours of release. It went on to top the album charts on both sides of the Atlantic and won a Grammy for Album of the Year. The album's first single, 'With Or Without You' reached Number One on the *Billboard* Hot 100 and Number Four in the UK. The band topped the US charts again with the second single, 'I Still Haven't Found What I'm Looking For', which peaked at Number Six in the UK.

While making the album, U2 continued to work with Brian Eno and Daniel Lanois, and also brought back former collaborator Steve Lillywhite to mix four songs. The opening track, 'Where The Streets Have No Name', was nearly dropped after its complex arrangement caused problems in the studio. It later became a Top 10 single in the UK and reached 13 in the US.

Around 20 tracks were recorded for *The Joshua Tree*, prompting thoughts of releasing a double album. A stronger single disc release was ultimately decided upon.

Number One singles:
US: I Still Haven't Found What I'm Looking For

Grammy awards: Album of the year; Best rock performance by a duo or group with vocal; Best performance music video

Label: US & UK: Island

Recorded in: Dublin, Ireland

Personnel:
Bono
The Edge
Adam Clayton
Larry Mullen Jr
Daniel Lanois
Brian Eno
Paul Barrett
Steve Lillywhite

Producer:
Daniel Lanois
Brian Eno

1   **Where The Streets Have No Name** (5:37)
2   **I Still Haven't Found What I'm Looking For** (4:37)
3   **With Or Without You** (4:56)
4   **Bullet The Blue Sky** (4:32)
5   **Running To Stand Still** (4:18)
6   **Red Hill Mining Town** (4:52)
7   **In God's Country** (2:57)
8   **Trip Through Your Wires** (3:32)
9   **One Tree Hill** (5:23)
10 **Exit** (4:13)
11 **Mothers Of The Disappeared** (5:14)

Total album length: 50 minutes

U2

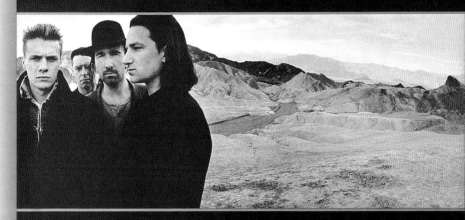

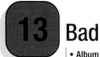

13 Bad

• **Album sales:** 11,900,000 | • **Release date:** August 1987 |

Following *Thriller*, Michael Jackson was arguably the biggest star in the world. However, the spectre of that album's enormous success made recording a follow-up something an unenviable task. With Quincy Jones and Jackson again co-producing, *Bad*, the resulting album, was a clear attempt to repeat the *Thriller* formula with a tougher edge. The title track was given a cinematic video, directed by Martin Scorsese, and starring Wesley Snipes alongside a newly leather-clad Jackson.

Once again Jackson managed to set new records when the debut single, 'The Way You Make Me Feel', became the first ever to enter the US chart in top position. Four more songs made it to the US Number One spot including 'Bad', 'The Way You Make Me Feel', 'Man In The Mirror', and ' Leave Me Alone'. In the UK, only 'I Just Can't Stop Loving You' topped the charts, but another three singles reached the Top Three.

The subsequent worldwide *Bad* Tour, which lasted from September 1987 until December 1988, brought in a gross revenue of $124 million.

Number One singles:
US & UK: I Just Can't Stop Loving You; US: Bad; Dirty Diana; The Way You Make Me Feel; Man In The Mirror

Grammy awards: None

Label: US & UK: Epic

Recorded in:
California, USA

Personnel:
Michael Jackson
Stevie Wonder
David Williams

Eric Gale
Steve Stevens
Bill Bottrell
Dann Huff
Michael Landau
Paul Jackson Jr
Larry Williams
Kim Hutchcroft
Gary Grant
Jerry Hey
John Barnes
Kevin Maloney
Jimmy Smith
Various other personnel

Producers:
Quincy Jones
Michael Jackson

1 Bad (4:06)
2 The Way You Make Me Feel (4:59)
3 Speed Demon (4:01)
4 Liberian Girl (3:53)
5 Just Good Friends (4:05)
6 Another Part Of Me (3:53)
7 Man In The Mirror (5:18)
8 I Just Can't Stop Loving You (4:10)
9 Dirty Diana (4:52)
10 Smooth Criminal (4:16)
11 Leave Me Alone (4:37)

Total album length: 48 minutes

Michael Jackson

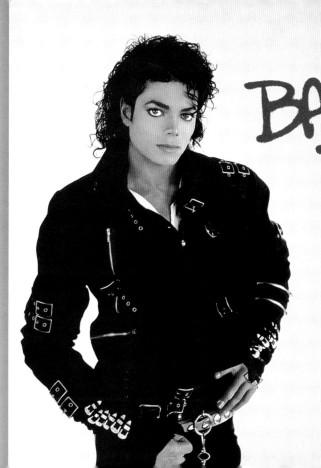

BAD

MICHAEL JACKSON

12 Slippery When Wet

| • **Album sales:** 12,900,000 | • **Release date:** August 1986 |

With only a few minor hits to their name, Bon Jovi had failed to scale the heights of rock stardom with their first two albums. The group therefore decided to tailor their third album into a surefire bestseller.

Bringing songwriter Desmond Child on board as a collaborator, the band put together a total of 30 songs which were then auditioned for focus groups consisting of teenagers from New York and New Jersey. Both the final selection and the running order were determined by the results from these auditions. The first choice of sleeve image (that of a busty woman clad in a wet T-shirt) was also ditched in favour of the inoffensive water-textured sleeve.

A further change in emphasis saw the single releases from the album supported by videos that tended to show off Jon Bon Jovi's pin-up good looks, bolstered by his carefully styled hair.

The resulting album, *Slippery When Wet*, became the biggest selling rock album of 1987 (though metal fans took exception to its pop-oriented content) and went multi-platinum. Two singles, 'You Give Love A Bad Name' and 'Livin' On A Prayer', reached Number One in the US (Number 14 and Number Four, respectively, in the UK) and Bon Jovi became one of the biggest rock acts in the world.

Number One singles:
US: You Give Love A Bad Name; Livin' On A Prayer

Grammy awards:
None

Label: US: Mercury; UK: Vertigo

Recorded in:
Vancouver, Canada

Personnel:
Jon Bon Jovi
Richie Sambora
Dave Bryan
Alec John Such
Hugh McDonald
Tico Torres
Bruce Fairbairn
Lema Moon
Tom Keenlyside

Producer:
Bruce Fairbairn

1 Let It Rock (5:25)
2 You Give Love A Bad Name (3:43)
3 Livin' On A Prayer (4:09)
4 Social Disease (4:18)
5 Wanted Dead Or Alive (5:09)
6 Raise Your Hands (4:17)
7 Without Love (3:31)
8 I'd Die For You (4:30)
9 Never Say Goodbye (4:49)
10 Wild In The Streets (3:56)

Total album length: 44 minutes

Bon Jovi

BON·JOVI

SLIPPERY WHEN WET

11 Dirty Dancing

| • **Album sales:** 12,500,000 | • **Release date:** September 1987 |

The impressive sales of the *Dirty Dancing* soundtrack were largely the result of the track (I've Had) The Time of My Life'. A duet sung by Jennifer Warnes and former Righteous Brother Bill Medley, the ballad reached Number One in the US, won a Grammy, and earned an Academy Award for Best Song. The single sold over 36,000,000 copies.

For such a huge success, the song had fairly inauspicious origins. Songwriter Franke Previte had recently been dropped by MCA when producer Jimmy Lenner invited him to write a song for *Dirty Dancing* (what Previte didn't know was that he was one of over 100 artists who had been extended the invitation). The filmmakers instantly realised that the submitted song was the perfect number for the final scene.

Other singles followed '(I've Had) The Time of My Life': 'Hungry Eyes', provided Eric Carmen with a Top Ten hit in the US while even the film's star, Patrick Swayze, hit the charts with 'She's Like the Wind'.

Number one singles:
US: (I've Had) The Time Of My Life

Grammy awards:
Best pop performance by a duo or group with vocal

Label: US & UK: RCA

Recorded in:
Various locations

Personnel:
Jennifer Warnes
Maurice Williams
Dr Robert
Tony Kiley
Mick Anger
Neville Henry

Bill Medley
Bruce Channel
Tom Johnston
Ronnie Spector
Estelle Bennet
Nedra Talley
Merry Clayton
Wendy Fraser
Patrick Swayze
Alfie Zappacosta
Maurice Williams
Various other personnel

Producers:
Peter Wilson
Michael Lloyd
Phil Spector
Leon Medica
Eric Carmen
Alfie Zappacosta

1 (I've Had) The Time Of My Life (Jennifer Warnes) (4:47)
2 Be My Baby (The Ronettes) (2:37)
3 She's Like The Wind (Patrick Swayze) (3:51)
4 Hungry Eyes (Eric Carmen) (4:06)
5 Stay (Maurice Williams & the Zodiacs) (1:34)
6 Yes (Merry Clayton) (3:15)
7 You Don't Own Me (The Blow Monkeys) (3:00)
8 Hey! Baby (Bruce Channel) (2:21)
9 Overload (Alfie Zappacosta) (3:39)
10 Love Is Strange (Mickey & Sylvia) (2:52)
11 Where Are You Tonight? (Tom Johnston) (3:59)
12 In The Still Of The Night (The Five Satins) (3:03)

Total album length: 39 minutes

Original Soundtrack

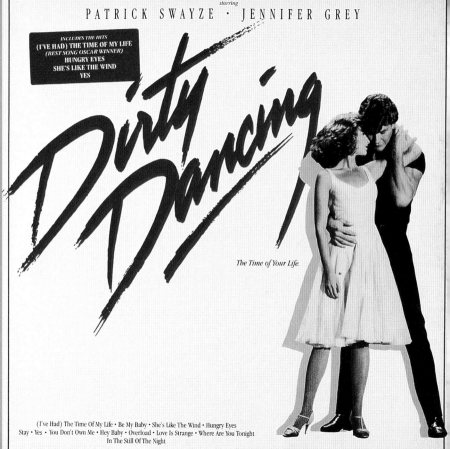

Selections From The Original Soundtrack From The Vestron Motion Picture
starring
PATRICK SWAYZE · JENNIFER GREY

INCLUDES THE HITS
(I'VE HAD) THE TIME OF MY LIFE
(BEST SONG OSCAR WINNER)
HUNGRY EYES
SHE'S LIKE THE WIND
YES

Dirty Dancing

The Time of Your Life.

Sleeve artwork by Pam Rodi and Adger Cowans

(I've Had) The Time Of My Life • Be My Baby • She's Like The Wind • Hungry Eyes
Stay • Yes • You Don't Own Me • Hey Baby • Overload • Love Is Strange • Where Are You Tonight
In The Still Of The Night

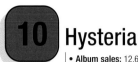

10 Hysteria

| • **Album sales:** 12,600,000 | • **Release date:** July 1987 |

Def Leppard had experienced their first taste of rock superstardom, albeit largely US-based, with the release of their 1983 album *Pyromania*. However, plans to build on this success proved problematic to say the least.

'Mutt' Lange declined an offer to produce the follow-up album, deciding to take a break after recording The Cars' *Heartbeat City*. Working instead with Jim Steinman, Def Leppard began recording tracks in Holland in 1984 before deciding that the producer's style wasn't appropriate for their music. At Lange's suggestion, the band instead turned to Nigel Green, who had been an engineer on their second album, *High'n'Dry*.

Then, on New Year's Eve, 1984, drummer Rick Allen lost his left arm in an automobile accident. He successfully learnt to use a custom-made drum kit, and rejoined Def Leppard in the studio in 1985. Lange came back on board, but was dissatisfied with the existing recordings and the album was started again, virtually from scratch.

Recording continued throughout 1986. *Hysteria* was finally released in 1987, but initial sales were slow and the first single, 'Women', failed to chart. Fortunes changed with the release of 'Animal', the second of the seven singles eventually released from the album.

Number One singles:
US: Love Bites

Grammy awards: None

Label: US: Mercury;
UK: Vertigo

Recorded in: Hilversum, Holland; Dublin, Ireland; Paris, France.

Personnel:
Joe Elliott
Steve Clark
Phil Collen
Rick Savage
Rick Allen

Producer:
Robert John 'Mutt' Lange

1 Women (5:41)
2 Rocket (6:34)
3 Animal (4:02)
4 Love Bites (5:46)
5 Pour Some Sugar On Me (4:25)
6 Armageddon It (5:21)
7 Gods Of War (6:32)
8 Don't Shoot Shotgun (4:10)
9 Run Riot (4:38)
10 Hysteria (5:49)
11 Excitable (4:19)
12 Love And Affection (4:35)

Total album length: 62 minutes

Def Leppard

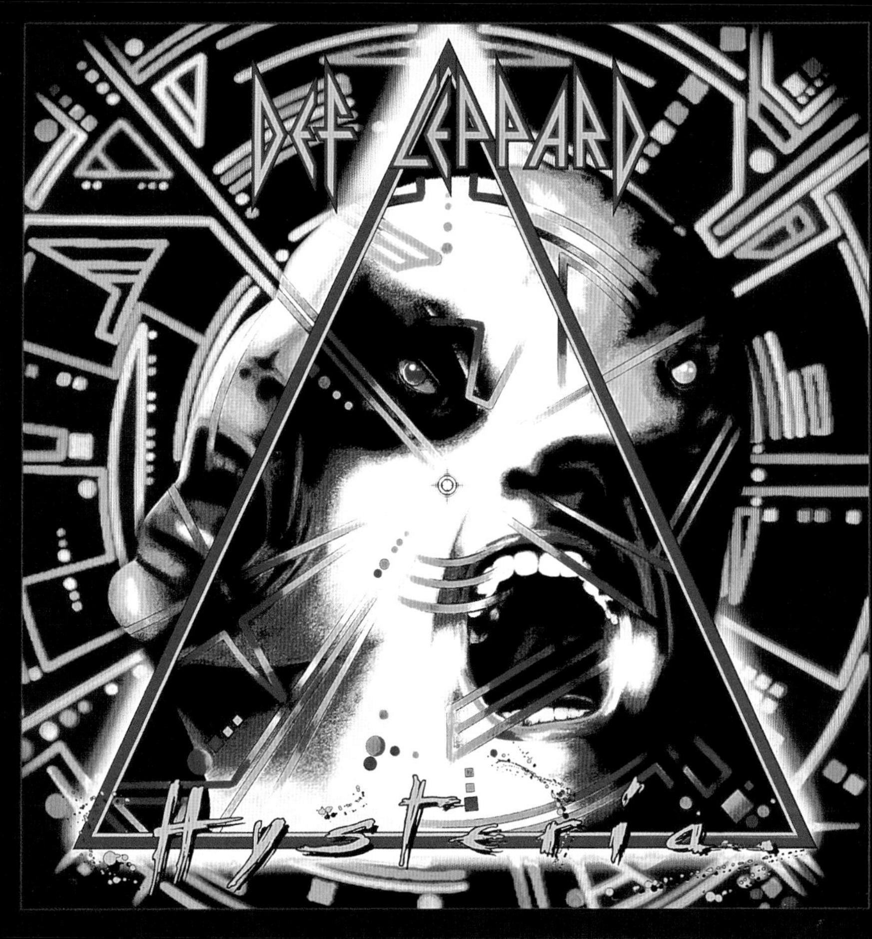

Sleeve artwork by Laurie Lewis and Ross Halfin

9 Brothers In Arms

| • **Album sales:** 12,900,000 | • **Release date:** May 1985 |

Dire Straits had spent some years building a reputation as expert musicians, solid songwriters and superb live performers. All this served as little warning of the impact that *Brothers In Arms* would have, both on the group's career, and on the public's regard for them. Bouyed by the Top 40 success of 'So Far Away', released earlier in the year, the album went platinum in the UK and entered the charts at Number One, a position it held for three weeks.

Much of the album's commericial success can be attributed to 'Money For Nothing', written by Mark Knopfler and Sting. Supported by a cutting-edge computer animated video, which guaranteed heavy rotation on the new music channels, the single reached Number One in the US and Number Four in the UK, won a Grammy for Best Music Video, and became the band's only million-selling single.

Other singles followed, including 'Walk of Life', which reached Number Seven in the US and Number Two in the UK. The song 'Brothers in Arms', while less successful on the charts, is remembered as having been the first CD-single to be sold commercially. With a pressing of only 400 copies, it has since become a sought-after collector's item.

Number One singles:
US: Money For Nothing

Grammy awards: Best music video, short form; Best rock performance by a duo or group with vocal

Label: US: Warner; UK: Vertigo

Recorded in:
Monserrat, West Indies; London, UK; New York, USA

Personnel:
Mark Knopfler
Hal Lindes
Guy Fletcher
Alan Clark
John Illsley
Terry Williams
Sting
Michael Becker
Randy Becker
Various other personnel

Producers:
Neil Dorfsman
Mark Knopfler

1 **So Far Away** (5:12)
2 **Money For Nothing** (8:26)
3 **Walk Of Life** 4:12)
4 **Your Latest Trick** (6:33)
5 **Why Worry** (8:31)
6 **Ride Across The River** (6:57)
7 **The Man's Too Strong** (4:40)
8 **One World** (3:40)
9 **Brothers In Arms** (6:59)

Total album length: 55 minutes

Dire Straits

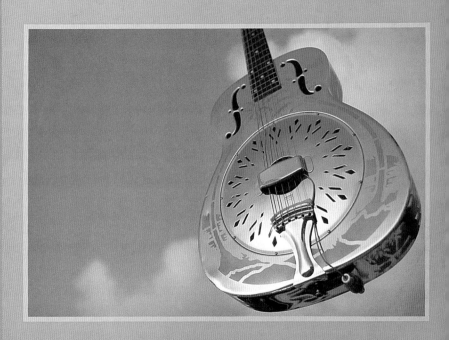

Sleeve artwork by Sutton Cooper

8 Live/1975-85

| • **Album sales:** 13,100,000 | • **Release date:** October 1986 |

Much of Bruce Springsteen's reputation, prior to the career turning point that was *Born in the U.S.A.*, had been built on the strength of his live shows, during which he regularly performed for over three hours. It was appropriate, then, that Springsteen would follow up his most successful album with a long-awaited live collection demonstrating the very strengths that had taken him to that point. Presented as a potted history of Springsteen's life and music over the previous decade, *Live/1975-85* starts with the relatively modest *Born To Run* tour and ends with his worldwide *Born In The U.S.A.* tour.

Despite it's ambitious breadth (no less than five LPs, 40 tracks, a three and a half hour running time) *Live/1975-85* debuted at Number One in the US album charts.

1   Thunder Road (5:41)
2   Adam Raised A Cain (5:25)
3   Spirit In The Night (6:22)
4   4th Of July, Asbury Park (Sandy) (6:29)
5   Paradise By The "C" (3:34)
6   Fire (3:12)
7   Growin' Up (7:57)
8   It's Hard To Be A Saint In The City (4:37)
9   Backstreets (7:27)
10 Rosalita (Come Out Tonight) (9:59)
11 Raise Your Hand (5:13)
12 Hungry Hearts (4:27)
13 Two Hearts (3:05)
14 Cadillac Ranch (4:50)
15 You Can Look (But You Better Not Touch) (3:51)
16 Independence Day (5:09)
17 Badlands (5:15)
18 Because The Night (5:18)
19 Candy's Room (3:09)
20 Darkness On The Edge of Town (4:24)
21 Racing In The Streets (8:13)
22 This Land Is Your Land (4:17)
23 Nebraska (4:16)
24 Johnny 99 (4:21)
25 Reason To Believe (5:19)
26 Born In The U.S.A. (6:07)
27 Seeds (5:11)
28 The River (11:37)
29 War (4:51)
30 Darlington County (5:12)
31 Working On The Highway (3:59)
32 The Promised Land (5:32)
33 Cover Me (6:58)
34 I'm On Fire (4:24)
35 Bobby Jean (4:26)
36 My Hometown (5:08)
37 Born To Run (5:02)
38 No Surrender (4:42)
39 Tenth Avenue Freeze-Out (4:18)
40 Jersey Girl (6:30)

Total album length: 216 minutes.

Number One singles:
None

Grammy awards: None

Label: US: Columbia; UK: CBS

Recorded in:
various locations

Personnel:
Bruce Springsteen

Nils Lofgren
Clarence Clemons
Roy Bittan
Danny Federici
Stan Harrison
Garry Tallent
Steve Van Zandt
Max Weinberg
Various other personnel

Producers:
Jon Landau
Chuck Plotkin

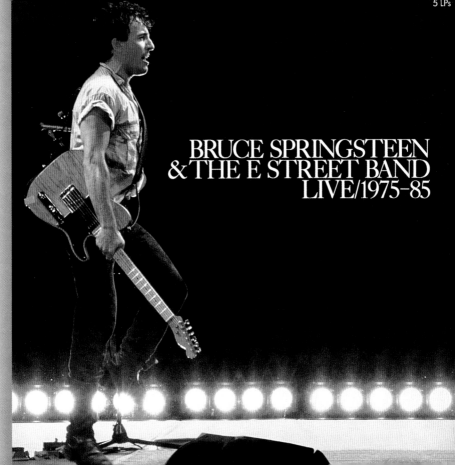

5 LPs

BRUCE SPRINGSTEEN
& THE E STREET BAND
LIVE/1975-85

Sleeve artwork by Sandra Choron and Neal Preston

7 Purple Rain

| • **Album sales:** 13,600,000 | • **Release date:** August 1984 |

Prince's previous album, *1999,* had brought the diminutive singer considerable success in the US, but it was his soundtrack to the 1984 hit film *Purple Rain* that was to make him and backing band The Revolution, into global superstars. The album spent 24 weeks at the top of the US album charts, reached Number Seven in the UK, and gave Prince his first two US Number One singles with 'When Doves Cry' and 'Let's Go Crazy'. The title track reached Number Two in the US, while 'I Would Die 4 U' and 'Take Me With U' charted in the *Billboard* Hot 100.

With a reputation for lyrical lewdness, the Prince retained his right to shock with tracks such as 'Darling Nikki', but there was a growing sense of maturity in the starkly arresting 'When Doves Cry'. The album won Prince two Grammy awards and an Academy Award for Best Song Score.

In addition to making the soundtrack, Prince took the starring role in *Purple Rain,* a loosely autobiographical film about a young Minneapolis rock musician struggling to make it big. The movie grossed over $5 million dollars at the box office and functioned as an extended promotional video for the album. Coupled with the record breaking success of his 1984–85 *Purple Rain* tour, the hype helped make the album into the biggest hit of Prince's career.

Number One singles:
US: When Doves Cry;
Let's Go Crazy

Grammy awards:
Best album or original score for a motion picture;
Best rock performance by a duo or group with vocal

Label: US & UK: Warner

Recorded in:
Los Angeles, USA

Personnel:
Prince
Wendy Melvoin
Lisa Coleman
Matt Fink
Brown Mark
Bobby Z
Apollonia
Novi Novog
David Coleman
Suzie Katayama

Producers:
Prince
The Revolution

1 Let's Go Crazy (4:39)
2 Take Me With U (3:54)
3 The Beautiful Ones (5:15)
4 Computer Blue (3:59)
5 Darling Nikki (4:15)
6 When Doves Cry (5:52)
7 I Would Die 4 U (2:51)
8 Baby I'm a Star (4:20)
9 Purple Rain (8:45)

Total album length: 44 minutes

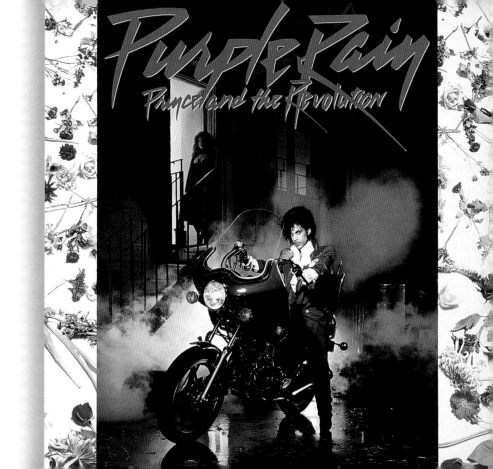

6 No Jacket Required

| • **Album sales:** 13,800,000 | • **Release date:** February 1985 |

Phil Collins had gradually established himself as a solo artist of note with two previous albums released outside the Genesis envelope. Although he remained insistent during the 1980s that he wasn't about to leave the group, *No Jacket Required* arrived during a period when Phil Collins was a far bigger name than Genesis. He was even able to recruit former Genesis frontman Peter Gabriel to perform backing vocals for 'Take Me Home', as well as Sting (on 'Long Long Way To Go', a song which Collins would perform to memorable effect at Live Aid).

The title was inspired after Collins was stopped from entering the bar at Chicago's Ambassador Hotel (where he was staying with Robert Plant) because his leather jacket wasn't deemed to be a 'proper' jacket.

The album won Collins the 1985 Grammy award for Album of the Year, affirming him as an artist with a fair degree of commercial clout, and consolidating his solo efforts alongside the respect he had already garnered for skills as both a producer and drummer. It reached the Number One spot in charts across the world, and spawned three hit singles, 'Sussudio', 'Take Me Home' and 'One More Night'.

Number One singles:
US: One More Night;
Sussudio

Grammy awards: Album of the year; Best male pop performance; Producer of the year (non-classical)

Label: US: Atlantic;
UK: Virgin

Recorded in:
London, UK

Personnel:
Phil Collins
Daryl Stuerner
Arif Mardin
The Phoenix Horns
Don Mynck
Lee Sklar
Helen Terry
Peter Gabriel
Sting
Various other personnel

Producers:
Phil Collins
Hugh Padgham

1 **Sussudio** (4:23)
2 **Only You Know And I Know** (4:20)
3 **Long Long Way To Go** (4:20)
4 **I Don't Wanna Know** (4:12)
5 **One More Night** (4:47)
6 **Don't Lose My Number** (4:46)
7 **Who Said I Would** (4:01)
8 **Doesn't Anybody Stay Together Anymore** (4:18)
9 **Inside Out** (5:14)
10 **Take Me Home** (5:51)
11 **We Said Hello, Goodbye (Don't Look Back)** (4:15)

Total album length: 50 minutes

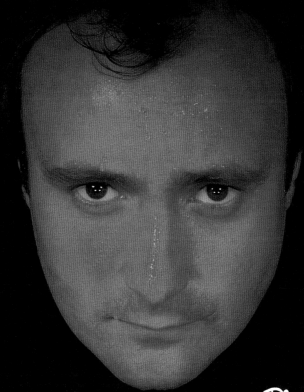

No Jacket Required

Phil Collins

5 Whitney Houston

| • **Album sales:** 14,200,000 | • **Release date:** February 1985 |

For an album that would hit the record books as the biggest selling debut by a female artist, *Whitney Houston* got off to an inauspicious start.

Houston had signed in 1983 to Arista, whose boss, Clive Davis, is commonly credited with discovering her. Davis was determined to make her debut album a success by recruiting only the best songwriters and producers for the task.

Despite Davis' enthusiasm many established producers were unwilling to throw their lot in with an unproven artist, and the album only started to get off the ground after Kashif came forward with a demo for 'You Give Good Love'. In the end, the label spent over $250,000 dollars in recording *Whitney Houston*, an unheard of amount for an artist's first recording.

Released on Valentine's Day, the album slowly built up momentum, reaching Number One spot later in the year, a position it held for 14 weeks. Such was its popularity that *Whitney Houston* was still the bestselling album in 1986, the year after its release.

Number One singles:
US & UK: Saving All My Love For You; US: How Will I Know; Greatest Love Of All

Grammy awards:
Best Female Pop Vocal Performance – Saving All My Love For You

Label: US & UK: Arista

Recorded in: N/A

Personnel:
Whitney Houston
Cissy Houston
Neil Vineberg
Paul Pesco

Ira Siegel
Corrado Rustici
Paul Jackson Jr
Kenny G
Vincent Henry
Jerry Hey
Marc Russo
Wayne Wallace
Robbie Buchanan
Preston Glass
Kashif
Teddy Pendergrass
Tom Scott
Various other personnel

Producers:
Narada Michael Walden
Kashif
Michael Masser
Jermaine Jackson

1 You Give Good Love (4:37)
2 Thinking About You (5:26)
3 Someone For Me (5:01)
4 Saving All My Love For You (3:58)
5 Nobody Loves Me Like You Do (3:49)
6 How Will I Know (4:36)
7 All At Once (4:29)
8 Take Good Care Of My Heart (4:16)
9 Greatest Love Of All (4:51)
10 Hold Me (6:00)

Total album length: 47 minutes

WHITNEY HOUSTON

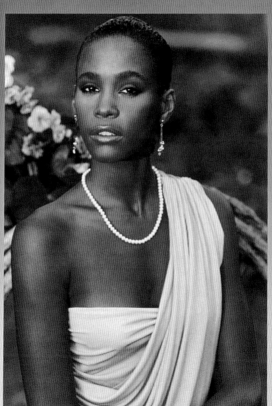

4 Appetite For Destruction

| • **Album sales:** 15,600,000 | • **Release date:** July 1987 |

Just as heavy metal seemed to be getting too long in the tooth to remain credible, Guns N' Roses arrived. The group successfully re-energised the genre with shameless gusto, and made the basic tenets of hard rock, as well as the accompanying attitude, fashionable once again.

Following an independent live EP release, Guns N'Roses were signed by Geffen in 1986, who launched their debut album, *Appetite For Destruction*, the following year.

Appetite For Destruction took its time to get noticed. Its potential for success was marred initially by the original sleeve, depicting a violent rape, which saw it banned by several major retailers. The cover was subsequently redesigned, and the album reissued.

'Welcome To The Jungle' started to get airplay on radio and TV music channels early in 1988 (and was also featured on the soundtrack of *The Dead Pool,* starring Clint Eastwood). However, it was 'Sweet Child O' Mine' which finally proved the album's selling point. The song was picked up by MTV and quickly made it to Number One in the US pop charts (although only 24 in the UK), helping the album to reach Number One in July 1988, a year after its release. 'Welcome To The Jungle' was subsequently re-released. A further single, 'Paradise City', made it into the Top Ten in the US and UK in 1989.

Number One singles:
US: Sweet Child O' Mine

Grammy awards:
None

Label: US & UK: Geffen

Recorded in:
California, USA

Personnel:
Axl Rose
Slash
Izzy Stradlin
Duff McKagan
Steven Adler

Producer:
Mike Clink

1 Welcome To The Jungle (4:32)
2 It's So Easy (3:21)
3 Nightrain (4:26)
4 Out Ta Get Me (4:20)
5 Mr. Brownstone (3:46)
6 Paradise City (6:45)
7 My Michelle (3:38)
8 Think About You (3:49)
9 Sweet Child O' Mine (5:54)
10 You're Crazy (3:16)
11 Anything Goes (3:25)
12 Rocket Queen (6:14)

Total album length: 53 minutes

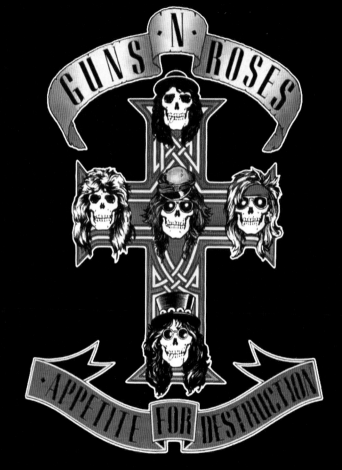

3 Born In The U.S.A.

| • **Album sales:** 15, 900,000 | • **Release date:** June 1984 |

Prior to the 1984 release of *Born In The U.S.A.*, Bruce Springsteen's career was qualified largely through strong reviews, healthy sales and a loyal following but he stopped short of unqualified mainstream stardom. Since the release of *Born To Run* in 1975, his songs had grown increasingly cynical and downbeat. Although *Born In The U.S.A.* continued this trend, its stadium-bound production helped create the Boss's greatest popular success. While commercially minded ears were drawn by the anthemic sound of singles like the title track, loyal fans were rewarded by songs that continued to focus on the working classes and the disenfranchised.

The first single, 'Dancing In The Dark', illustrated most startlingly how Springsteen was broaching new musical ground with its keyboard hook, while the video was famously responsible for making a star out of Courtney Cox.

Although *Born In The U.S.A.* failed to yeild any number one singles, seven of twelve tracks went on to become Top Ten hits in the US, while the album itself stayed in both the US and UK charts for more than two years.

Number One singles:
None

Grammy awards:
Best male rock vocal performance – Dancing In The Dark

Label: US: Columbia; UK: CBS

Recorded in:
New York, USA

Personnel:
Bruce Springsteen
Steve Van Zandt
Clarence Clemons
Danny Federici
Roy Bittan
Garry Tallent
Max Weinberg
La Bamba
Ruth Jackson
Richie Rosenberg

Producers:
Bruce Springsteen
Jon Landau
Chuck Plotkin
Steve Van Zandt

1 **Born In The U.S.A.** (4:39)
2 **Cover Me** (3:26)
3 **Darlington County** (4:48)
4 **Working On The Highway** (3:11)
5 **Downbound Train** (3:35)
6 **I'm On Fire** (2:36)
7 **No Surrender** (4:00)
8 **Bobby Jean** (3:46)
9 **I'm Goin' Down** (3:29)
10 **Glory Days** (4:15)
11 **Dancing In The Dark** (4:01)
12 **My Hometown** (4:33)

Total album length: 46 minutes

BORN IN THE U.S.A./BRUCE SPRINGSTEEN

2 Back In Black

| • **Album sales:** 19,100,000 | • **Release date:** July 1980 |

The February 1980 death of AC/DC's lead singer, Bon Scott, came close to curtailing the rock band's recent rise to international status. Nevertheless, with a new singer, Brian Johnson, and the recently recruited Robert John 'Mutt' Lange continuing on production, AC/DC managed a return to the record shelves just five months later with their biggest album. *Back In Black* was certified platinum within two months of release and transformed AC/DC into one of the biggest rock groups in the world.

Lange, brought on board for the previous album, *Highway To Hell*, had managed to fine tune the band's raucous hard rock sound into something altogether more viable commercially and approaching the anthemic at times.

Meanwhile, Brian Johnson proved not only a capable match for Bon Scott on vocals, but in many ways surpassed the late singer.

A number of the album's strongest tracks, 'Rock & Roll Ain't Noise Pollution' and 'You Shook Me All Night Long', enjoyed success in the singles charts, while 'Hell's Bells' became something of a signature track.

The massive sales of *Back In Black* also prompted the American release of the band's 1976 album *Dirty Deeds Done Dirt Cheap*, which had been previously available only in Europe and, in a different form, Australia.

Number One singles:
None

Grammy awards:
None

Label: US & UK: Atlantic

Recorded in:
Nassau, Bahamas

Personnel:
Brian Johnson
Angus Young
Malcolm Young
Cliff Williams
Phil Rudd

Producer:
Robert John 'Mutt' Lange

1 Hells Bells (5:09)
2 Shoot To Thrill (5:14)
3 What Do You Do For Money Honey (3:33)
4 Given The Dog A Bone (3:30)
5 Let Me Put My Love Into You (4:12)
6 Back In Black (4:13)
7 You Shook Me All Night Long (3:28)
8 Have A Drink On Me (3:57)
9 Shake a Leg (4:03)
10 Rock & Roll Ain't Noise Pollution (4:12)

Total album length: 42 minutes

AC/DC

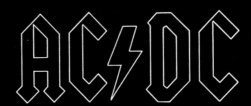

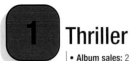

1 Thriller

| • **Album sales:** 29,300,000 | • **Release date:** December 1982 |

Michael Jackson had already released one career-defining solo album with the Quincy Jones production *Off the Wall*. This, nevertheless, did little to prepare the world for the behemoth that was 1982's *Thriller*. The album had it all: rock, soul, pop, Jackson's distinctive vocals, and a celebrated selection of collaborators.

Number One singles:
US & UK: Billie Jean;
US: Beat It

Grammy awards:
Album of the year; Record of the year – Beat It; Best male pop vocal performance – Thriller; Best male rock vocal performance – Beat It; Producer of the year; Best male R&B vocal performance – Billie Jean; Best R&B Song – Billy Jean; Best Video Album

Label: US & UK: Epic

Recorded in:
California, USA

Personnel:
Michael Jackson
Paul McCartney
Vincent Price
Eddie Van Halen
Janet Jackson
LaToya Jackson
James Ingram
Dean Parks
David Foster
Larry Williams
Jerry Hey
David Paich
Various other personnel

Producers:
Michael Jackson
Quincy Jones
Brian Banks

The first single, 'The Girl Is Mine', reached the Top Ten on both sides of the Atlantic, but it was the ambitious videos for 'Billie Jean' and 'Beat It' that would provide the foundation for the album's success. Thanks in part to Eddie Van Halen's powerhouse guitar solo, 'Beat It' was readily embraced by MTV, making Jackson the first black artist to find success on the network. Equally, Jackson's star power helped gain an extensive audience for the new channel.

An unprecedented seven of the album's nine tracks became Top Ten hits in the US. The success of *Thriller*, and the impact of the videos, redefined expectations within the music industry for ever.

1 **Wanna Be Startin' Somethin'** (6:02)
2 **Baby Be Mine** (4:20)
3 **The Girl Is Mine** (3:42)
4 **Thriller** (5:57)
5 **Beat It** (4:17)
6 **Billie Jean** (4:57)
7 **Human Nature** (4:05)
8 **P.Y.T. (Pretty Young Thing)** (3:58)
9 **The Lady In My Life** (4:57)

Total album length: 42 minutes

Michael Jackson

Michael Jackson
Thriller

includes
THE GIRL IS MINE
BILLIE JEAN
BEAT IT

Appendix: Facts and figures

The 20 highest-ranking US artists (position on list given in brackets)

1 Michael Jackson: *Thriller* (1)
2 Bruce Springsteen: *Born In The USA* (3)
3 Guns N' Roses: *Appetite For Destruction* (4)
4 Whitney Houston: *Whitney Houston* (5)
5 Prince & The Revolution: *Purple Rain* (7)
6 Bon Jovi: *Slippery When Wet* (12)
7 Madonna: *Like a Virgin* (16)
8 Lionel Richie: *Can't Slow Down* (17)
9 Van Halen: *1984* (19)
10 REO Speedwagon: *High Infidelity* (24)
11 Garth Brooks: *Garth Brooks* (25)
12 Beastie Boys: *Licensed To III* (26)
13 Journey: *Escape* (27)
14 ZZ Top: *Eliminator* (28)
15 New Kids On The Block: *Hangin' Tough* (30)
16 Billy Joel: *An Innocent Man* (31)
17 Bobby Brown: *Don't Be Cruel* (33)
18 Paula Abdul: *Forever Your Girl* (34)
19 Tracy Chapman: *Tracy Chapman* (35)
20 Eagles: *Live* (37)

The 20 highest-ranking international artists

1 AC/DC: *Back In Black* (2)
2 Phil Collins: *No Jacket Required* (6)
3 Dire Straits: *Brothers In Arms* (9)
4 Def Leppard: *Hysteria* (10)
5 U2: *The Joshua Tree* (14)
6 George Michael: *Faith* (15)
7 The Police: *Synchronicity* (29)
8 Genesis: *Invisible Touch* (36)
9 INXS: *Kick* (42)
10 Whitesnake: *Whitesnake* (47)
11 Foreigner: *4* (5)
12 Peter Gabriel: *So* (56)
13 Tears For Fears: *Songs From The Big Chair* (57)
14 Men At Work: *Business As Usual* (62)
15 Enya: *Watermark* (66)
16 Sade: *Diamond Life* (67)
17 Wham!: *Make It Big* (68)
18 Milli Vanilli: *Girl You Know It's True* (71)
19 Fleetwood Mac: *Tango In The Night* (74)
20 Bryan Adams: *Reckless* (85)

The 10 highest-ranking solo artists

1 Michael Jackson: *Thriller* (1)
2 Bruce Springsteen: *Born In The USA* (3)
3 Whitney Houston: *Whitney Houston* (5)
4 Phil Collins: *No Jacket Required* (6)
5 George Michael: *Faith* (15)
6 Madonna: *Like A Virgin* (16)
7 Lionel Richie: *Can't Slow Down* (17)
8 Garth Brooks: *Garth Brooks* (25)
9 Billy Joel: *An Innocent Man* (31)
10 Bobby Brown: *Don't Be Cruel* (33)

The 10 highest-ranking bands

1 AC/DC: *Back In Black* (2)
2 Guns N' Roses: *Appetite For Destruction* (4)
3 Prince & The Revolution: *Purple Rain* (7)
4 Dire Straits: *Brothers In Arms* (9)
5 Def Leppard: *Hysteria* (10)
6 Bon Jovi: *Slippery When Wet* (12)
7 U2: *The Joshua Tree* (14)
8 Van Halen: *1984* (19)
9 REO Speedwagon: *Hi Infidelity* (24)
10 Beastie Boys: *Licensed To Ill* (26)

Record labels with the most albums in the Top 100

1 Columbia (13 Albums)
2 Atlantic (10 Albums)
3 Geffen (10 Albums)
4 Warner (10 Albums)
5 CBS (9 Albums)
6 Capitol (7 Albums)
7 Epic (7 Albums)
8 Virgin (7 Albums)
9 Mercury (6 Albums)
10 Vertigo (6 Albums)
11 MCA (5 Albums)
12 A&M (4 Albums)
13 Motown (4 Albums)
14 Sire (4 Albums)
15 Arista (3 Albums)
16 Elektra (3 Albums)
17 Portrait (3 Albums)
18 Island (2 Albums)
19 Music For Nations (2 Albums)
20 RCA (2 Albums)
21 Riva (2 Albums)
22 WEA (2 Albums)

Artists with the most albums in the Top 100
(artists ranked by number of albums and aggregate score of album positions)

1 Madonna:
Like A Virgin (16)
True Blue (21)
Madonna (61)
Like A Prayer (65)

2 Bruce Springsteen:
Born In The USA (3)
Live 1975–1985 (8)
The River (77)

3 Phil Collins:
No Jacket Required (6)
Face Value (44)
But Seriously (45)

4 AC/DC:
Back In Black (2)
Who Made Who (79)
For Those About To Rock (98)

5 Lionel Richie:
Can't Slow Down (17)
Dancing On The Ceiling (88)
Lionel Richie (90)

6 Michael Jackson:
Thriller (1)
Bad (13)

7 Whitney Houston:
Whitney Houston (5)
Whitney (18)

8 Def Leppard:
Hysteria (10)
Pyromania (23)

9 Bon Jovi:
Slippery When Wet (12)
New Jersey (32)

10 U2:
The Joshua Tree (14)
Rattle And Hum (48)

11 Billy Joel:
An Innocent Man (31)
Glass Houses (41)

Appendix

Albums containing the most Number One singles

1 *Bad*: **Michael Jackson**
5 Number Ones: US & UK: I Just Can't Stop Loving You; US: Bad; Dirty Diana; The Way You Make Me Feel; Man In The Mirror

2 *True Blue*: **Madonna**
5 Number Ones: US & UK: Papa Don't Preach; US: Live To Tell; Open Your Heart; UK: True Blue; La Isla Bonita

3 *Whitney*: **Whitney Houston**
4 Number Ones US & UK: I Wanna Dance with Somebody (Who Loves Me); US: Didn't We Almost Have It All; So Emotional; Where Do Broken Hearts Go

4 *Make it Big*: **Wham!**
4 Number Ones: US & UK: Wake Me Up Before You Go-Go; Careless Whisper; US: Everything She Wants; UK: Freedom

6 *Faith*: **George Michael**
4 Number Ones: US: Faith; Father Figure; Monkey; One More Try

7 *Forever Your Girl*: **Paula Abdul**
4 Number Ones: US: Forever Your Girl; Straight Up; Opposites Attract; Cold Hearted

Albums that have won the most Grammys

1 Michael Jackson: *Thriller* (8 Grammys)
2 Christopher Cross: *Christopher Cross* (5 Grammys)
3 Phil Collins: *No Jacket Required* (3 Grammys)
4 Tracy Chapman: *Tracy Chapman* (3 Grammys)
5 Bonnie Raitt: *Nick Of Time* (3 Grammys)
6 Tina Turner: *Private Dancer* (3 Grammys)
7 Prince & The Revolution: *Purple Rain* (2 Grammys)
8 Dire Straits: *Brothers In Arms* (2 Grammys)
9 U2: *The Joshua Tree* (2 Grammys)
10 The Police: *Synchronicity* (2 Grammys)
11 Paul Simon: *Graceland* (2 Grammys)
12 U2: *Rattle & Hum* (2 Grammys)
13 Anita Baker: *Rapture* (2 Grammys)
14 Original soundtrack: *Flashdance* (2 Grammys)
15 Original soundtrack: *Miami Vice* (2 Grammys)

Soundtrack albums in the Top 100

1 *Purple Rain:* Prince (7)
2 *Dirty Dancing:* Various Artists (11)
3 *Top Gun:* Various Artists (20)
4 *Footloose:* Various Artists (22)
5 *The Big Chill*: Various Artists (55)
6 *The Jazz Singer*: Neil Diamond (63)
7 *Flashdance*: Various Artists (76)
8 *Who Made Who*: AC/DC (79)
9 *Miami Vice*: Various Artists (95)

Index